SECRETS OF
NATIVE AMERICAN
HERBAL REMEDIES

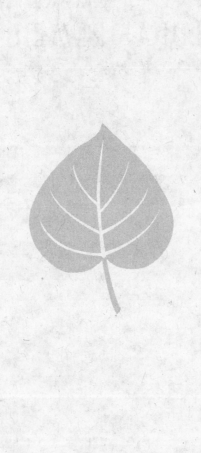

SECRETS OF NATIVE AMERICAN HERBAL REMEDIES

A Comprehensive Guide to the Native American
Tradition of Using Herbs and the Mind/Body/Spirit
Connection for Improving Health and Well-Being

ANTHONY CICHOKE, D.C., PH.D.

AVERY
A MEMBER OF PENGUIN PUTNAM INC.
NEW YORK

Every effort has been made to ensure that the information in this book is complete and accurate. However, neither the publisher nor the author is engaged in rendering professional advice or services to the individual reader. The ideas, procedures, and suggestions in the book are not intended as a substitute for consulting with a physician. All matters regarding health require medical supervision. Neither the author nor the publisher shall be liable or responsible for any loss, injury, or damage allegedly arising from any information or suggestion in this book.

The recipes contained in this book are to be followed exactly as written. Neither the publisher nor the author is responsible for specific health or allergy needs that may require medical supervision or for any adverse reactions to the recipes contained in this book.

Most Avery books are available at special quantity discounts for bulk purchase for sales promotions, premiums, fund-raising, and educational needs. Special books or book excerpts also can be created to fit specific needs. For details, write Putnam Special Markets, 375 Hudson Street, New York, NY 10014.

a member of
Penguin Putnam Inc.
375 Hudson Street
New York, NY 10014
www.penguinputnam.com

Library of Congress Cataloging-in-Publication Data

Cichoke, Anthony J.
Secrets of Native American herbal remedies : a comprehensive guide
to the Native American tradition of using herbs and the mind/body/spirit
connection for improving health and well-being / Anthony Cichoke.
p.   cm.
Includes bibliographical references and index.
ISBN 1-58333-100-X
1. Herbs—Therapeutic use.   2. Indians of North America—Medicine.
3. Spiritual healing.   I. Title.
RM666.H33 C585   2001   00-068258
615'.321'08997—dc21

Printed in the United States of America

15 17 19 20 18 16

Book design by Jill Weber

THIS BOOK IS DEDICATED TO THE MEMORY OF *Vern "Sonny" Johnson, Jr.* He was a Native American, a member of the Lummi Nation, a talented woodcarver, and a dedicated fighter for improved water quality. When diagnosed with stomach cancer, Vern returned to the old traditional ways of healing, integrating them into his therapy program. He turned to herbal medicines and American Indian remedies (including the sweat lodge) and spent four days at New Mexico's Ojo Caliente Hot Springs, soaking in and drinking the healing waters. Vern never gave up, and he lived years longer than the few weeks predicted by practitioners of organized "conventional" medicine. He was a hero and a credit to his family, the Lummi Nation, Native Americans, and all humankind. By returning to the old ways of his people, he showed us how to fight illness and extend life . . . with dignity.

Thank you, Vern, it was an honor knowing you. I dedicate this book to you and to each person's search for the true dignity of life.

CONTENTS

Acknowledgments

I'd like to thank the following individuals and institutions for their encouragement, cooperation, informational materials, and assistance in helping to complete this book: James R. Bowman, Ruby Windspirit, the DeGalger Library (Southern Methodist University), Daniel Gagnon, Paula Wallis, Armand Minthorn, E. Thomas Morning Owl, the Confederated Tribes of the Umatilla Indian Reservation, Althea Wolf, Tamas Tslikt Cultural Institute, Michael Moore, Steven Dentali, Phyllis Hogan, Donna Chesner, D. E. Moerman, Malissa Minthorn, Carl and Bobbi Sampson, Anita Paz, Cecilia Carpenter, Edward Alstat, Rick Stewart, Big Dave Archambault, Wilfred Klingsat, Wilmer Mesteth, Birgil Kills Straight, James Duke, Little Dave Archambault II, Jewell James, Vern Johnson, the Lummi Indian Nation, Northwest Indian College, Nancy Carroll, Kenny Cooper, Henry M. Cagey, Ruth and Ted Solomon, Tom Edwards, Cynthia Wilson, Sid Williams, Florence Kinley, Chip Richie, Steven Heape, Rich-Heape Films, Inc., Roger Canard, Freita Kelliche, Indian Country Today, Rita White Butterfly, Helen Felix Baco, Kevin Peniski, Jeff Schiller, National College of Naturopathic Medicine Library, Eclectic Library, Eclectic Institute, Life University, Cleveland Chiropractic College, David Schiller, Rod Jones, Jan Nicholas, Janet Zand, Beatriz Steeghs, Tierona Low Dog, Shirley Hankins-Carlisle, the American Indian Chamber of Commerce of Texas, the Confederated Tribes of Warm Springs, Oregon, and Katie Cichoke and William Cichoke.

A huge thanks goes to the helpful employees of the libraries of America and especially of the West Slope Library in Portland, Oregon, for their hard work and never-ending cooperation.

Special thanks to Norman Goldfind and Rosa Goldfind for their constant help, and to my secretary, Mrs. Karen Hood, for all of her assistance in the preparation of this book, including research, typing, and editing. Thanks also to proofreader Beata Szewezk, to Dara Stewart and Laura Shepherd at Avery for their special work as editors, and to John Duff for his support.

Finally, my eternal thanks to my wife, Margie, for her continuous assistance and for enduring the mountains of paper in our house these past three years.

PREFACE

This American Indian herbal book gives you simple, yet effective herbal remedies to fight specific health conditions. With a brand-new approach to traditional information, this book shows you how to help yourself and how to take charge of your life.

Until quite recently, most Americans believed that only prescription drugs, surgery, chemicals, radiation, or some other "scientific" treatment—administered and sanctioned by a medical doctor—could cure illness or injury. But sadly, this crisis approach has resulted in a failing health-care system with skyrocketing costs. In 1960, our national health expenditures were 5 percent of the gross national product (GNP). By 1990, that figure exceeded 12 percent, and by 1996, health expenditures amounted to more than 13.6 percent of the GNP. That equates to over one trillion dollars, and it's still climbing! Sadly, modern health care is so expensive that it's not uncommon for a family to lose their life savings fighting a serious medical condition—even if they're fortunate enough to have health insurance. Today's orthodox health care is too impersonal and too expensive. It stresses crisis therapy (rather than prevention) and offers questionable results. In fact, on a per-capita basis, the present U.S. health-care system costs more than any other in the world but ranks only thirty-seventh in terms of quality of care, according to an analysis by the World Health Organization.

More and more people are actively looking for alternatives to orthodox medicine. People are returning to their roots, back to traditional health care.

And in so doing, they are finding effective ways of healing—naturally. As with the American Indians, who learned how to help themselves, people are learning how to walk in harmony with nature, and how to balance their lives. They are also learning the importance of believing in the power of the Creator.

How striking that with the most advanced medical system in the world, the most exotic drugs, the best and most expensive equipment, and the most advanced surgical techniques available anywhere, people are returning to the old traditional ways in hordes. People are looking beyond "the establishment" for health care. In fact, in the past year, some 50 percent of all adults between the ages of thirty-five and forty-nine have used some form of alternative health care. In 1997, Americans made approximately 629 million visits to alternative medicine practitioners, including herbalists, chiropractors, naturopaths, homeopaths, acupuncturists, and spiritual healers. In fact, more people visited alternative health-care practitioners than visited conventional primary-care physicians! Isn't the use of the term *alternative* ironic, then? After all, what we now call "alternative" is actually thousands and thousands of years old. It would seem to me that "modern," orthodox medicine should be called alternative instead.

The times are changing in the medical community as well. More and more doctors, scientists, and healers are integrating alternative or complementary (adjunctive) medicine and therapies into their practices. Organized medicine is beginning to view alternative methods and traditional herbal medicine more seriously. In fact, the *Journal of the American Medical Association* devoted an entire issue to alternative medicine (November 18, 1998).

Alternative health care is nothing new to me; I learned it, quite literally, at my father's knee. My father, Dr. Anthony J. Cichoke, Sr., was the first chiropractor to receive a license from the state of Illinois. For more than forty years, I watched my father heal people by employing many of the practices used effectively by the American Indians. He combined a body, mind, and spirit approach to healing, saying a prayer before treating each patient, then laying on hands, and adjusting the patient. In addition, he suggested herbs and other nutrients, as well as healing therapies that would help improve the patient's condition. My father drew on information he had obtained from Native American tribes while growing up in Wisconsin, from information from his football days with Jim Thorpe (the famous Native American football player), and from experiences in central Illinois. My father helped many people, as evidenced by the long lines of patients that formed down the outer hall from his office.

From an early age, "traditional healing" was my way of life. However, when my dad was alive, herbal remedies and other alternative therapies, such as chiropractic, were considered "quackery." In fact, many orthodox physicians would cross to the other side of the street rather than pass by my father. Yet, he received many secret referrals from a wide variety of confident orthodox medical doctors and even from the famous Mayo Clinic.

Personally, I continued to follow the path taught me by my father and practiced chiropractic for some twenty-five years, employing many of the healing techniques used by Native Americans and by my father. From my father, I learned that symptoms are a reflection of disorder, of disturbed energies in the whole body, a sign that the body—mentally, physically, and nutritionally—is out of balance. For these reasons, it was quite natural for me to write about Native American healing, which follows the same principles and emphasizes balancing the body, not just treating symptoms.

Through years of research and writing, I have discovered that Native American healing concepts share many healing principles with other traditional methods of healing, such as traditional Chinese medicine, Tibetan medicine, Ayurvedic medicine, Eastern-European folk medicine, Celtic healing, African healing, and so on. The use of herbs, the belief in the importance of balance and harmony in the body, the concept of treating the whole person (not just a collection of symptoms), a close connection with nature, and the belief in a Creator—a power far greater than any one of us—all seem to be at the heart of these ancient healing arts.

One of the fastest-growing segments of alternative health care is the use of herbs to treat illness. Just check the growing amount of shelf space devoted to various herbs in your local grocery store, health-food store, and drug store. Surveys by *Prevention* magazine and NBC News indicate that over 70 million Americans now use herbal medicines to treat illness and to maintain health.

Herbal healing, of course, is nothing new; it's been around for thousands of years. Herbs were the first drugs and the primary medicine used by humans everywhere. Native Americans learned to use herbs empirically; that is, by trying them and observing their effects on the body. They also watched the animals, realizing that if an herb worked for an animal, it might work for humans, too. Over the centuries, they learned which herbs worked for which conditions. Modern research has verified the efficacy of many of the herbs traditionally used by Native Americans. In fact, isolated compounds from many of those herbs are now used as the basis for modern medicine.

This book divulges the secrets of Native American herbal healing remedies. Today, the public is bombarded with mountains of information on healing, nutrition, and herbs. This deluge of information is often contradictory, misleading, confusing, and discouraging—not to mention overwhelming. This book cuts through the volumes of hype and gives you concise and useful information to integrate Native American herbal healing secrets into your daily life and help you better fight disease and injuries.

We all can profit from the vast knowledge and wisdom acquired by Native Americans. They can teach us much if we would only look, listen, try to understand, and follow their examples. This book will show you how. 🐦

PART ONE

Native American Herbs

Native Americans have used herbs medicinally for thousands of years. The first written record of the herbs they used and how they used them begins only with the first contact between Europeans and the tribes, including the Wampanoag, that inhabited the eastern shore of North America. Unfortunately, no written records of herbal use exist before that time to document exactly when they began healing with herbs. As Europeans immigrated to the New World and as settlers traveled across the plains, the Native Americans taught them how to get well and stay well using nature's medicines. The knowledge the Native Americans have shared with them has given us a rich heritage of healing. In fact, it is believed that at least two hundred of our modern prescription medicines were derived from Native American herbs. Today, synthetic duplications of natural herbal compounds, as well as naturally grown herbs themselves, account for numerous over-the-counter medicines.

What Is an Herb?

What is an herb? It depends on whom you ask. Some say an herb must have a woody stem and be used as medicine or flavoring. Well then, that eliminates many plants and bushes without woody stems. Others say an herb is an herbaceous but not a woody plant. So bushes and trees don't count. For the purposes of this book, we consider an herb any useful plant having medicinal properties.

Native American Herb Use

Native Americans learned which herbs were good for which conditions empirically, often through trial and error. They tried an herb, and if the patient felt better, then they might use that herb again. A plant's color, shape, odor, and taste also greatly influenced its application. For example, red plants were good for the blood, yellow plants were used to treat jaundice. Plants that looked like the liver were used to treat liver problems. This philosophy of using similar shapes and colors is called the "doctrine of signatures" and is found in the traditional healing art of many cultures. This doctrine is a belief that a plant's physical appearance can reveal its therapeutic benefits. For example, ginseng (*Panax quinquefolium*) is shaped like male genitalia and was used as an aphrodisiac and to improve sexual potency. The East Coast tribes, including the Delaware, used ginseng to increase male fertility. Sometimes, use of an herb for a particular condition was prompted by a vision or a dream. In fact, a medicine man might experiment with a certain herbal medicine or combination for some time after being given the knowledge in a dream. Another frequently used method of finding herbs was observing the animals to see which herbs they ate.

There are hundreds of Native American herbal cures and more than enough information to substantiate their outstanding healing capabilities. For example, Daniel A. Moerman, ethnobotanist and author of *Native American Ethnobotany,* documents 24,945 plants used therapeutically by the Native Americans. Therefore, needless to say, this book cannot possibly include every healing plant. Instead, we have tried to include those herbs that have historically been used most frequently to treat the conditions listed in Part Three of this book.

In discussing the healing herbs used by the Native Americans, the supernatural beliefs of Native American culture must first be emphasized. These beliefs are tightly, intricately, and unchangeably woven into the tapestry of a Native American's daily life. It is the combined healing of the spirit, heart, and mind that makes medicine work. For native peoples, the word *medicine* does not simply describe some physical thing such as a capsule, pill, potion, lotion, or powder (or even surgery); it also speaks of the greater "power" behind the cure.

The Native American Ritual of Gathering Herbs

It is this spiritual belief that dictates the procedures and ceremonies that are to be followed when herbs and other plants are gathered. Phyllis Hogan, the founder and director of the Arizona Ethnobotanical Research Association, works with a total of sixteen Native American tribes, including the Navajo and Hopi. She is an applied ethnobotanist who has worked in Arizona for nearly thirty years, documenting comparative plant uses among the state's indigenous people. She also owns the Winter Sun Trading Company, a Flagstaff company specializing in traditional herbs and American Indian art. An expert in the use of southwestern botanicals and the first person to receive the honorary position of practitioner associate in anthropology from North Arizona University, Phyllis was taught by the Navajo to always pick herbs early in the morning and begin by burning juniper, smudging some of the soot on your skin, and praying to the sun deity. Then, she makes a prayer offering of cornmeal to the plant, telling it her name and that she wants to use the plants to heal. She then asks permission to pick the plant's fellow plants and waits for the plant to give permission. According to Phyllis, "This can be in the form of a vibratory connection between the picker and the plants; perhaps the wind blows or you get an intuitive feeling or hear songs. And if the plant does not give permission, you do not pick that day. You don't pick the plant you are praying to, because it is your emissary to the plant world. You then give an offering to the earth, then the sky, then the four directions, starting with the east and going clockwise. And also honor the middle. We also put a little cornmeal on our heads. This is a connection to the spirit world and also a sign of purity." She adds that some plants don't want to come, some pull easily and some won't. It is also important to never take more than you need and always leave at least one-fourth of what's there. Rare and endangered plants should never be picked, and you should never pick in someone else's picking place. Some areas have been picked for thousands of years by the same clan members. Pickers show respect for the plant world, always wearing nice clothing and jewelry when gathering herbs. This is because they are meeting the deities and want to be recognized as someone of stature. Phyllis's favorite pastime is herb-gathering because she stops thinking of worldly problems during this time.

According to Phyllis, pickers only pick one type of plant per day. "This is because you must take responsibility for the plant and feed it with cornmeal or pollen again, then pray to welcome it." Once the plants are picked they are placed on clean sheets or other cloths and aligned with the herb, roots, leaves, and flowers pointing in the same direction as the other herbs, roots, leaves, and flowers. They are then fed cornmeal once again and welcomed, and told again why they are needed. They are then allowed to rest for a day; only one species of plant is picked a day. Before preparing the herbs, they are again prayed to and thanked for being here. Only then are they prepared into tinctures, extracts, or other forms.

Additional Herb Uses

In addition to their medicinal and food uses, Native Americans have used the plants that grow wild in the fields and forests for weaving, dyeing, basket-making, and for making brushes, ropes, cords, pottery, and decorations. They have used herbs as hunting charms or basket charms and as flavorings and spices.

Herbs were also used in sacred ceremonies, to purify shamans, and to assist in visions and dreams. For example, the great Sioux medicine man and chief, Sitting Bull, had a vision three weeks before the Battle of Little Bighorn that all the white soldiers would fall in defeat and his people would triumph. This is, of course, exactly what happened when Custer and his men met Sitting Bull in battle.

Tobacco was one of the most important herbs for many tribes. It can have both positive and negative effects. According to the Traditional Native American Tobacco (TNAT) Seed Bank and Education Program, "When used improperly, such as when it is smoked in cigarettes, or otherwise ingested in a commercial form, tobacco is a deadly killer. When used properly, in very small amounts in traditional Native American ceremonies and prayer, tobacco (like sacramental wine in a Catholic mass) becomes a positive source of religious power." In addition to tobacco, herbs used in sacred ceremonies and pipe ceremonies include sage, lobelia, gentian, myrtle, magnolia, and slippery elm.

Herbs were of particular benefit in clearing the mind and soul and warding off evil spirits. When used in this way, herbs were often burned in smudges, bundles of herbs that are burned much like incense. Some of the most popular purifying herbs used to please the spirits and the human senses were aromatic, including cedar, juniper, mesquite, pinion, red willow, sage, and sweet grass. Herbs were also smoked for pleasure, as well as for fighting respiratory disorders. A few herbs used for these purposes include angelica, bearberry, corn silk, coltsfoot, dogwood, deer's tongue, mullein, sumac, valerian, and yerba sante.

As mentioned earlier, herbs are used in sweat lodges to detoxify and cleanse the body. Native Americans have also used herbal mixtures in enemas to stimulate the removal of unwanted toxins through perspiration, bowel excretion, urination, or vomiting. In fact, Virgil Vogel, author of *American*

Indian Medicine, notes that American Indians actually discovered the bulb syringe and the enema tube, using fish and animal bladders plus inserts constructed from reed and small hollow bones. These Native American techniques were successfully used for centuries and are still in use today. Today, Navajo medicine leaders claim they can even cure people with cancer using routine colon cleansing and fasting, accompanied by sweating.

Enemas used by the Native Americans void the body of undesirable toxins trapped in the intestines and also purify the body spiritually. Maintenance of a healthy colon is essential for optimal body balance. The Native Americans have also used herbal laxatives to purge deadly toxins and as a preventive measure against illness. Enemas can be administered at home, or colonic therapy can be performed under the guidance of a trained chiropractor or naturopath.

My Enzyme Kidney Flush and Enzyme Toxin Flush are excellent companions to American Indian cleanses. See my book *The Complete Book of Enzyme Therapy* for a complete description of both flushes.

A Return to Natural Ways

Today, there is a revival of herbal medicine, a movement back to the natural ways. Most, if not all, of these people are paying for herbal cures out of their own pockets, with no insurance reimbursement. Many people feel closer to the earth, to nature, and to the Creator when they are using herbs. Further, herbs and natural healing are less expensive than orthodox medicine. With skyrocketing health-care costs, inexpensive but effective herbal healing seems an increasingly welcome alternative. In addition, most of the time herbs do not cause the serious side effects that so often accompany the use of pharmaceuticals.

For many years, the American Medical Association (AMA) was very much against many herbal remedies, labeling herbal use and other "alternative" treatments as quackery. Fortunately, even their views are changing.

The World Health Organization (WHO—an agency of the United Nations created to develop global health standards) is encouraging all countries to promote and adopt the use of traditional medicines, such as herbs, to ensure the survival and increased use of traditional methods. This is primarily an economic decision since drugs may cost up to $4 a pill or more, and who in a less affluent country (and perhaps even in a more affluent country like the United States) could afford taking these tablets two or three times per day? In contrast, herbs can actually be grown locally in the wild and harvested. In many instances, herbal cures can be just as effective as expensive pharmaceuticals.

There are a number of valuable books available for information on gathering, growing, and storing herbs. If you are gathering herbs, however, respect the plants, as Native Americans do. They have always known that as long as they respect nature, nature will care for their needs. Unfortunately, many people are not that considerate. Several herbs that used to grow extensively in North America are now threatened and may become extinct because of overzealous herbalists.

Although there is a wealth of herbal knowledge present within the culture of American Indians, it is not always easy to encourage Native Americans to part with their herbal secrets. Many feel that Native Americans have been exploited enough through the centuries, and they do not want to perpetuate that exploitation. Others believe that the power of their healing systems might be weakened by sharing them with non-Indians, who might misrepresent the techniques. Many of the sacred songs and healing rituals were passed on during vision quests or initiations into secret societies; so naturally, Native Americans are not comfortable sharing this fragile, sacred information with those who might alter it or abuse it—especially when most who hold the knowledge had to undergo so much in order to attain it. Fortunately, however, there are those who believe that sharing Native American healing secrets with non-Native Americans is the only way to keep them alive and protect them from extinction. This, then, is my goal: to celebrate the greatness of the Native American herbal healing traditions and to share this information with you so that you can take charge of your life for better health.

Healthful Constituents of Herbs

For centuries, Native Americans have used whole herbs for the treatment of disease; and while they knew that the herbs worked, it wasn't always known why. For example, teas of pine needles or rose hips were used to cure colds or flu. As we now know, it was the vitamin C and bioflavonoids in the pine needles and rose hips that possessed the healing action. Today, science is identifying the healing properties contained in herbs, including vitamins, minerals, enzymes, and phytochemicals.

PHYTOCHEMICALS

Phytochemicals are the naturally occurring chemicals found in plants ("phyto" means plant). These plant nutrients can be isolated and concentrated from herbs and other plants.

Some phytochemicals are effective as cancer fighters or antioxidants; others lower cholesterol, decrease plaque in the arteries, stimulate immune system function, or stimulate enzyme production. Following are some of the phytochemicals found in many of the herbs used by American Indians over the centuries.

Alkaloids

Alkaloids are found in a number of plants, including goldenseal. They prevent the overgrowth of yeast in the body, maintaining healthy levels of bacteria in the gastrointestinal and urinary tracts; and they support immune function.

Anthocyanidins

Anthocyanidins are a class of phytochemicals that are found in bilberries, black currants, and raspberries. They fight free radicals (a by-product of metabolic reactions in the body that can lead to such degenerative illnesses as cardiovascular disease and cancer); reduce blood-vessel plaque formation, maintaining blood flow and reducing the risk for cardiovascular disease; inhibit edema (swelling due to fluid accumulation); fight inflammation; and improve vision.

Chlorophyll

Chlorophyll is found in all green herbs. It fights bacteria, helps in the healing of burns and wounds, and fights cancer. It is also an excellent source of vitamin K.

Diterpenes

Diterpenes are found in many herbs, including rosemary. It is a potent antioxidant, anticancer agent, and anti-liver-toxin agent.

Eleutherosides

Eleutherosides are found in Siberian ginseng. They increase stamina, stimulate appetite, and increase physical and mental vigor. They stimulate metabolism, the immune system, and the central nervous system. Eleutherosides are also helpful in combating some of the problems of menopause, including irregular periods and hot flashes.

Essential Fatty Acids

Essential fatty acids, namely omega-3 and omega-6 fatty acids, are fats that are essential to good health but cannot be made by the body. They maintain the integrity of cell membranes and of myelin sheaths (the protective covering of nerve fibers). They stimulate the production of prostaglandins (hormonelike substances that mediate metabolism, smooth-muscle activity, and nerve transmission, among other functions), lower blood cholesterol levels, and strengthen immunity. They can be found in many herbs, including saw palmetto.

Flavonglycosides

Flavonglycosides are potent antioxidants (fighters of free radicals). They also dilate blood vessels, improving blood flow; improve mental clarity; improve vision and hearing; and help alleviate depression. They are found in *Ginkgo biloba.*

Gingerols

Gingerols are antioxidants and improve digestion of proteins and fats. They also soothe the stomach and fight liver toxicity and inflammation. They are the active constituents of ginger.

Ginkolic Acid

Ginkolic acid, found in *Ginkgo biloba,* is yet another antioxidant. It improves circulation and mental clarity, treats depression, and fights cancer.

Glycyrrhizins

Glycyrrhizins, the protective phytochemicals found in licorice, have anti-viral, anti-inflammatory, and skin-protective properties. They also inhibit tumor formation.

Hesperidin

Hesperidin, found in milk thistle seeds, is an antioxidant that protects capillaries and strengthens cell membranes. It works well against liver disease and protects against ultraviolet rays.

Hypericin

Hypericin is the active component of St. John's wort. It helps improve mood, possibly by regulating neurotransmitters in the brain.

Isothiocyanates

Isothiocyanates are found in horseradish. They induce the production of protective enzymes and inhibit DNA damage, thereby reducing the risk for breast cancer.

Lactones

Lactones, found in kava kava root, protect the body against cancer by eliminating carcinogens.

Lipoic Acid

Lipoic acid, found in many plant foods, is a potent antioxidant that eliminates heavy metals from the body, protects against cancer and heart disease, normalizes blood-sugar levels, and slows aging. Lipoic acid is a key factor in energy production.

Phenolic Acids

Phenolic acids are antioxidants that inhibit the formation of nitrosamines (cancer-causing agents). They are found in berries, parsley, and all flowering plants.

Phthalides

Phthalides, found in parsley, detoxify carcinogens and stimulate the production of beneficial enzymes.

Polyacetylenes

Polyacetylenes also are found in parsley. They regulate the production of prostaglandins and protect against carcinogens.

Proanthocyanidins

Proanthocyanidins, found in elderberry and bilberry, are another class of antioxidants. They protect against cancer, high blood-cholesterol levels, and the influenza virus. They also strengthen blood-vessel walls.

Quercetin

Quercetin is a flavonoid that is widely distributed in the plant kingdom. (Flavonoids are naturally occurring antioxidants found in many fruits, vegetables, and other plants.) Quercetin has antihistamine, anti-inflammatory, and anticancer properties. It also stabilizes cell membranes and reduces capillary fragility.

Rosemarinic Acid

Rosemarinic acid is the active constituent of rosemary. It fights nausea, intestinal gas, and indigestion. It is also effective against headaches.

Salin

Salin, or salicin, is found in white willow bark. It fights inflammation, relieves pain and fever, and fights the influenza virus.

Saponins

Saponins, found in ginseng root, licorice, black cohosh, yucca, and many other herbs, fight cancer formation, enhance wound healing, and reduce cholesterol levels. They have anti-inflammatory, antibacterial, and antifungal properties.

Silymarin

Silymarin is the active constituent of milk thistle. It is an antioxidant and protects the liver.

Tannins

Tannins are widely distributed in plants. They are antioxidants that have antiviral properties and strengthen capillaries. They protect against cancer, heart disease, and asthma.

Terpenes

Terpenes (the common name for monoterpenes) are antioxidants found in *Ginkgo biloba*.

Triterpenoids

Triterpenoids prevent dental decay and fight ulcers, cancer, and liver toxicity. They are found in licorice root and gotu kola.

ENZYMES

Enzymes are present in all herbs that have not been exposed to high temperatures or to alcohol during preparation. The presence of enzymes is essential in order to activate the phytochemicals and other nutrients in the herbs. Enzymes also are very important for improving the absorption, action, and bioavailability of these herbs in the body. If enzymes have been destroyed during the processing of the herbal preparation, it is important to take enzyme supplements in addition to the herbs. Enzyme supplements should contain a combination of proteases (enzymes that work on proteins), lipases (break up fats), and amylases (break up carbohydrates).

Using Herbs

The herbs, plants, and roots American Indian ancestors gathered for healing were often used fresh, sometimes dried, and sometimes ground into powders. They were used individually or combined to make teas, poultices, or potions to heal various diseases. Herbs can be used in a variety of ways.

COMPRESSES

Compresses are used for topical applications and are made by soaking cloth strips in a hot herbal solution and then placing the cloth directly on the affected area of the body. To avoid blistering or other injury, always test a warm compress, making sure it is not too hot before applying to the skin. Compresses are very effective in treating muscle strains and ligament sprains.

DECOCTIONS

Herbal decoctions are teas made from the bark, berries, leaves, roots, or seeds of the plant. Decoctions are usually made by simmering the herb for about twenty to thirty minutes, although some barks and roots may require an hour. To make a decoction: Place two ounces of fresh herbal roots, twigs, bark, and/or stems (if using dried herbs, use only one ounce) in an ovenproof glass pot, add four cups of cold filtered or distilled water, and simmer until the liquid decreases in volume to two cups. Strain liquid into a tea cup or serving container.

ESSENTIAL OILS

Essential oils are extracted from herbs by steam distillation or cold pressing. They may *not* be taken internally, and, because they are very strong, they should be diluted in a carrier oil before being placed on the skin.

INFUSIONS

An infusion is a tea made by steeping (not boiling) the buds, flowers, leaves, or other parts of the plant for several minutes in hot water. The difference between a decoction and an infusion is that the herbs are simmered to make a decoction and steeped to make an infusion. Remember, the longer a preparation steeps, the more phytochemicals will be extracted from the herb. In addition, the longer it steeps, the more tannins will be extracted and the more bitter the taste will be. To make an infusion: Place one ounce of dried, or two and one half ounces of fresh, herbs (leaves, flowers, etc.) in a pint of distilled, filtered, or fresh boiling water, and steep about five to ten minutes (some herbs take longer than others; see discussions of specific herbs in this section for guidelines). Strain. A typical dose would be half a cup three times per day.

OINTMENTS AND SALVES

Ointments and salves are prepared by mixing herbal teas, extracts, or powders with petroleum jelly or some other oily or fatty base. They are applied directly to the skin. To make an ointment: Place three ounces of fresh (or two ounces of dried) herbs in a one-quart ovenproof glassware pot. Add one cup of pressed sunflower-seed oil or almond oil and heat the oil until very hot or just below the simmering point (be careful to prevent the oil from burning and/or igniting). Because the herbs contain moisture, they may "pop" while simmering in the oil. Use caution to prevent getting burned. Place the mixture in an oven for two hours at 170° F. Remove from the oven and let cool. Strain the mixture off into sterile bottles. If you'd like, you can add an additional sprig of the herb to each bottle; however, this will only make the presentation prettier, it will not improve the medicinal properties of the salve. Use topically as needed. Adding one ounce of beeswax to the strained liquid will make the ointment more solid when it cools to room temperature.

POULTICES

Poultices are hot, moist herbal concentrations made by placing herbs on a loose cloth such as muslin which is then applied directly to the skin. (Compresses, by contrast, are made by soaking cloth strips in an herbal solution.) Poultices are frequently used to treat inflammations. To make a poultice: Fill a square of cheesecloth with boiled or steeped herbs. The liquid from the herbs will moisten the cheesecloth. Apply while warm (as hot as can be tolerated). Discard any cooled poultice (when reheated, medical properties are not restored). Suggestion: Make two poultices; when one cools, the second can be placed on the affected area and the first discarded.

POWDER

Powdered herbs are made by drying the herbs and grinding, chopping, or crushing them. The resulting powder can be placed in capsules or formed into tablets. The powder can also be used to make a tea.

SYRUP

To produce an herbal syrup, add herbs or herbal teas to a sugar or honey solution and boil to thicken. To make syrup: Heat one cup of a fresh decoction or infusion. Add one cup of raw maple syrup, sugar, or honey and stir until the sweetener is dissolved. Cool, then pour into dark, amber-colored bottles, and store. A typical dose would be one teaspoon three times a day. *Note:* Honey will help preserve the syrup, while giving it a more palatable taste. Syrups are often easier to swallow than tablets or capsules and are of particular benefit for those suffering from a sore throat, cold, or cough, as syrups tend to coat the throat.

TINCTURES

Herbal tinctures are prepared by adding alcohol to dried or fresh herbs. To make a tincture: Pour two cups of 40-percent (80-proof) grain alcohol, such as brandy or vodka, over two ounces of fresh herbs or one ounce of dried herbs. Do not use metal or plastic. Store in a cool, dark place for two weeks (shake daily). After two weeks, strain the mixture, squeezing the herbs. Store in an amber dropper bottle. A typical dose would be one teaspoon, or twenty drops (under the tongue), three times per day.

VINEGARS

Herbal vinegars are flavorful additions to many foods and also can be used medicinally. To make an herbal vinegar: place herbs (two tablespoons or more) in a wide-mouth jar with a sealable lid. Pour one pint of apple-cider, malt, or rice vinegar over the herbs. The strength of the herbal vinegar will vary according to the amount of herbs used. Our purpose here is to impart beneficial phytochemicals rather than flavor. Allow the vinegar to stand in a dark, cool place for two weeks (the longer the herbs remain in the vinegar, the more they will flavor the solution). A typical dose would be one teaspoon, or twenty drops (under the tongue), three times per day.

Choosing the Herbs That Are Right for You

Choosing an herb or herbal combination is not always easy. There are many factors to consider when choosing the herb that is best for you. In addition to fresh and dried herbs, herbs are also available in capsules. Check the label on the bottle for your first clues in deciding to purchase an herbal product. Also make sure that the label provides directions for use, the weight of the ingredients in milligrams, an expiration date, and price. It's also important that the label provides the percentage of the marker compound present. For example, with St. John's wort, one must make sure to buy a standardized formulation with .3 percent hypericum.

Taking Herbal Supplements

Take the herbs as indicated on the label of the bottle or as directed by a well-trained alternative health-care practitioner in order to minimize any potential side effects. If you are taking herbs to improve digestion, take them thirty minutes or just before your meals. If you are fighting a disease or disorder, take the herbs between meals. Be aware of any side effects that your herbal supplements may cause, and advise your alternative health-care practitioner if any occur.

Storing Herbal Supplements

Keep your herbs and herbal supplements stored in a cool, dry place with the bottle top firmly tightened.

THE HERBS

THE HERBS IN THIS SECTION are presented alphabetically by common name of the herb. The genus and species are also listed to help clarify the exact herb discussed. There can be a great deal of confusion in discussing a particular herb because herbs were so often named after the condition or symptom they treated, rather than by any scientific method. For instance, any herb that treats a lung condition was often called lungwort. So the herb that the Native Americans in Florida referred to as lungwort might be a totally different herb from what other tribes in other parts of the country might call lungwort. This, of course, has led to an abundance of confusion, not only among the casual herb user but also among "expert" herbologists.

Note: Many herbs are known to be dangerous for pregnant women. Others may be safe. It is my opinion, however, that no pregnant woman should use herbs of any kind without the recommendation and knowledge of a well-trained metabolic health-care practitioner.

Agrimony

Agrimony (*Agrimonia* sp.) is a perennial herb found all over the world and goes by many names, including cockleburr, sticklewort, stickwort, burr marigold, and liverwort. Native Americans have used primarily two types of agrimony—*Agrimonia eupatoria* and *Agrimonia gryposepala*. It can help relieve skin, mouth, and throat inflammations and has been used to treat colds and asthma. Agrimony is an astringent, so it makes an effective antidiarrheal agent, a fact that several tribes, including the Cherokee and the Iroquois, have discovered. The Cherokee have also used agrimony to normalize the bowels, treat fever, ease hunger pangs in children, and build up the blood. Other uses for this herb include treating snake bites, jaundice, gout, and worms. When applied topically, agrimony leaves can help draw out thorns and splinters, stop cuts from bleeding, and help heal eczema, skin wounds, and sores.

To make a tea from agrimony, pour one cup of boiling water over two to four teaspoons of dried agrimony leaves or any of the aerial (aboveground) parts of the plant. Let steep for fifteen minutes. Strain. Take one tablespoon at a time, up to one cup per day. Agrimony is bitter tasting, so you may want to sweeten with honey.

Caution: Agrimony may increase your sensitivity to sunshine. It also contains tannins, which, if taken in amounts greater than three grams per day, can cause constipation and other digestive problems.

See also ALLERGIES; BITES AND STINGS, INSECTS; CATARRH; COUGHS AND COLDS; DIARRHEA; GOUT; INTESTINAL WORMS; *and* PNEUMONIA *in Part Two.*

Alumroot

The root of the Heuchera plant, called alumroot (*Heuchera Americana*) is an astringent used by the Cherokee, Blackfoot, Menominee, Navajo, Shuswap, and others to treat diarrhea and other gastrointestinal complaints. At one time (1820-1882), alumroot was listed as an official drug in the *United States Pharmacopoeia*, a book published by the United States Food and Drug Administration (FDA) every five years that lists all of the drugs approved for use by the FDA. When applied topically, compresses made with alumroot can help relieve hemorrhoid pain and help heal sores, wounds, and bites.

To prepare a tea from alumroot, pour one cup of boiling water over about an inch-long piece of the dried root. Let steep for thirty minutes. Strain. Take one to two tablespoons up to four times daily.

To make a compress, soak strips of cloth in the alumroot tea. Apply the compress to the affected area until the compress cools.

See also DIARRHEA *in Part Two.*

Angelica

The angelica plant, also called masterwort, alexanders, and archangel, is a perennial, aromatic plant that grows to be anywhere from two to eight feet tall. Native Americans have used many types of angelica, including *Angelica atropurpurea* (purple angelica), *A. arguta*, *A. pinnata*, *A. lucida*, and *A. archangelica*, to treat primarily colds and stomach disorders including diarrhea, gastritis, gas, and dyspepsia. Angelica also makes an effective diuretic and appetite stimulant.

Angelica infusions were used by the Iroquois in steam baths to treat headaches and frostbite. Angelica root poultices were applied to broken bones, and angelica tea served as a topical treatment for ulcers. Angelica was also widely used as a purification herb, added to sacred pipes and burned in healing ceremonies.

To make a tea, pour one cup of boiling water over two teaspoons of crushed angelica seeds. Let steep for thirty minutes. Strain. Take two tablespoons up to four times a day. If using angelica root, place two teaspoons of dried angelica root in a pan with three cups of water. Bring to a boil, then reduce heat and simmer until the liquid is reduced to one and a half cups. Remove from the heat and strain. Take a quarter cup up to four times daily.

Caution: Angelica appears to cause photodermatitis, an allergic skin reaction to the sun, so stay out of the sun if you are using this herb. Avoid angelica if you are pregnant, as it is a uterine stimulant.

See also CANCEROUS TUMORS; DIARRHEA; FATIGUE; FLATULENCE; HEARTBURN; *and* INDIGESTION *in Part Two.*

Balsam Fir

The balsam fir (*Abies balsamea*) is native to the northeastern United States and adjacent Canada where it is used principally for paper pulp and lumber and as a source of the liquid resin called Canada balsam. The balsam fir has erect cones and flattened needlelike leaves. In the eastern United States, it is commonly used as a Christmas tree.

Native Americans utilize the needles, resin, roots, branches, and bark from the balsam fir. Many tribes, including the Algonquin, Woodlands Cree, Iroquois, Menominee, Micmac, Ojibwa, and Potawatomi treat colds with a tea made from the sap or bark. The Ojibwa also inhale the smoke from the needle-like leaves to treat colds.

The gum of the fir makes an effective treatment and also a protective coating for burns, wounds, and cuts. The Chippewa inhale steam created by melting balsam gum to relieve headaches, while the Iroquois have used the steam created from a decoction of the branches to relieve rheumatism and as an aid to childbirth.

To make a tea, cover one teaspoon of the bark with two cups of water in a pan and bring to a boil. Boil for thirty minutes and strain. Take a quarter cup a day.

See also Arthritis; Sore Throat; *and* Tonsillitis *in Part Two.*

Barberry

Barberry (*Berberis vulgaris*) is a deciduous bush (also called pipperidge bush and berberry) that can grow up to ten feet in height. It is related to Oregon grape (see Oregon grape in this section). Tea made from the barberry fruit or the root bark is used to treat fever, sore throats, diarrhea, and intestinal disorders. Barberry contains an alkaloid called berberine, which has demonstrated significant antimicrobial activity against bacteria, fungi, protozoans, and viruses. A root decoction makes an effective topical wash for cuts and bruises.

Native Americans made good use of the barberry bush. The berries were eaten raw or made into jam, the root was used raw or boiled as a flavoring and in stew, and the wood and the bark make a yellow dye.

To prepare tea from the berries, pour one cup of boiling water over one to two teaspoons of the ripe berries (either whole or crushed). Let steep for fifteen minutes and then strain. If using barberry roots, place half a teaspoon of the dried and powdered root bark in a pan with one cup of water. Bring to a boil and boil for twenty to thirty minutes. Remove from the heat, cool, and strain. You may want to sweeten with honey. Drink up to one cup per day of the tea, one tablespoon at a time.

Caution: An overdose of the root bark can cause diarrhea, kidney irritation, light stupor, nosebleeds, and vomiting.

See also ABSCESS; ALLERGIES; ANEMIA; BACK PAIN; BOILS; CANKER SORES; DIARRHEA; FATIGUE; GOUT; HANGOVER; HEARTBURN; INDIGESTION; PSORIASIS; *and* TUBERCULOSIS *in Part Two.*

Bayberry

Also called American bayberry and wax myrtle, bayberry (*Myrica cerifera*) is an evergreen shrub or small tree that can grow as high as thirty-five feet. Bayberry is also called candleberry and waxberry because the wax from the berries has been used to make candles. An infusion from the dried root bark is used to treat coughs and colds. The Mohegans have treated kidney disorders with such a tea. Native Americans have also used bayberry to treat influenza, scurvy, stomach cramps, and gynecological problems.

A wash made from the root bark is effective in treating skin infections, diseases, and ulcers, perhaps because bayberry contains a chemical called myricitrin, which has antibiotic properties. Bayberry is very high in selenium, as well as in calcium, chromium, iron, manganese, sodium, and vitamin C.

To make a tea, place one teaspoon of the powdered root bark in a pan, cover with two cups of water, and bring to a boil. After boiling for fifteen minutes, remove from the heat and let cool. Skim off the wax, and strain. The taste will be bitter, so you may want to sweeten with honey. Take one to two cups per day, a few swallows at a time.

See also COLITIS; HANGOVER; HEARTBURN; INFLUENZA; MALAISE; NAUSEA AND VOMITING; SINUSITIS; SORE THROAT; TONSILLITIS; *and* TOOTHACHE *in Part Two.*

Bee Balm

Bee balm (*Monarda fistulosa*), also called wild bergamot and Oswego tea, is an aromatic perennial herb that grows up to three feet in height. Many tribes, including the Blackfoot, Chippewa, Crow, Flathead, Lakota, Meskwaki, Navajo, Ojibwa, and Teton Sioux, have used bee balm tea to treat coughs and colds, fever, and abdominal pains, including those caused by flatulence. The Menominee have also used the leaves and flowers to make a tea to treat catarrh.

The Winnebago apply boiled leaves of bee balm topically to treat acne and skin eruptions. Kiowas soothed insect bites and stings by applying a mixture of crumpled bee balm leaves, spotted bee balm (*Monarda pectinata*), and saliva.

To make a tea, pour one cup of boiling water over one teaspoon of bee balm leaves. Let steep for thirty minutes and strain. Take one to two cups per day, half a cup at a time.

See also CATARRH; FLATULENCE; *and* NAUSEA AND VOMITING *in Part Two.*

Betony

Betony (*Stachys officinalis*) is a perennial herb, also called purple betony, lousewort, and wood betony, that can grow up to about two feet in height. Betony is an effective muscle relaxant and is also used to treat a number of conditions, including asthma, bronchitis, heartburn, bladder and kidney problems, and intestinal worm infestations. Topically, the plant juice is used to heal cuts, sores, and skin ulcers.

To make a tea, pour one cup of boiling water over one to two teaspoons of betony leaves or other aerial parts. Let steep for thirty minutes and strain. Take up to two cups per day, one tablespoon at a time.

Caution: Avoid this herb if you are pregnant, as it stimulates the uterus.

See also NERVOUSNESS *and* STRESS *in Part Two.*

Big Sagebrush

Big sagebrush (*Artemisia tridentata*) is a shrub that can grow up to fifteen feet in height but is usually three to ten feet. It has been widely used by numerous tribes in the West to treat colds and gastrointestinal complaints, including diarrhea. Recent research indicates big sagebrush also has antifungal activity.

Native Americans have long used big sagebrush as a seasoning and a fiber to make thatch and linings for shoes, in addition to using it for its medicinal value. They have also woven clothing from the bark.

To make a tea, pour one cup of water on one to two teaspoons of sagebrush root. Let soak for eight hours. Strain. Take two to four tablespoons a day.

Caution: Avoid this herb if you are pregnant.

See also ATHLETE'S FOOT; CANDIDIASIS; SPRAINS AND STRAINS; *and* THRUSH *in Part Two.*

Bilberry

Bilberry (*Vaccinium myrtillus*) is a perennial shrub closely related to the blueberry. Also known as whortleberry, blaeberry, and windberry, the bilberry plant grows about eighteen inches tall and produces blue-black berries. The berries have a long history of use in treating diarrhea, respiratory problems, and gastrointestinal problems. Bilberry has also been used to treat fever. Native Americans have used it as a gargle for sore throats and as a wash for sores, ulcers, and wounds. Bilberry contains chemicals that protect and strengthen the blood vessels that feed the eyes, so it is an important herb in fighting macular degeneration (see this condition in Part Three). Bilberry also is very high in iron, manganese, phosphorus, and zinc; and high in magnesium, potassium, selenium, thiamin, vitamin A, and vitamin C.

To make a tea, place one teaspoon of the dried berries in a glass container and cover with one cup of water. Let soak overnight. Take one cup per day.

See also ARTHRITIS; CATARRH; MACULAR DEGENERATION; *and* SPRAINS AND STRAINS *in Part Two.*

Black Cohosh

Also known as black snakeroot, squawroot, and rattleroot, black cohosh (*Cimicifuga racemosa*) is a tall (up to nine feet high) perennial herb that is native to the United States and Canada. The root of this plant (dried and fresh) is probably best known for treating menopausal symptoms such as hot flashes, but it also promotes menstruation and relieves menstrual pain and amenorrhea (cessation of periods). In fact, between 1820 and 1936, the *United States Pharmacopoeia* listed black cohosh as an effective means to promote menstruation and as a sedative for rheumatism. Modern research indicates that black cohosh is a safe and effective alternative to estrogen replacement therapy, commonly prescribed for menopausal women. According to E. Thomas Morning Owl of the Confederated Tribes of Umatilla, Oregon, *cohosh* means "breast" in Umatilla.

In addition to its value for treating gynecological problems, black cohosh has been used by Native Americans as a sedative, a diuretic, an anticonvulsive, and as treatment for high blood pressure, as well as a number of respiratory conditions, including pleurisy, pneumonia, asthma, and croup. The Nanticoke Indians (from Delaware and eastern Maryland) used the root to make a tonic, while the Winnebago drank a decoction made from this plant to relieve rheumatism. The Cherokee used black cohosh in many ways: as a sedative, a tonic, and a diuretic, and to treat respiratory problems and rheumatism. The Iroquois used it as a blood purifier and to promote the flow of milk in nursing mothers.

It can also be used in steam baths as a treatment for rheumatism. A poultice made by pounding the leaves can be applied to sore backs. Black cohosh is very high in selenium and high in chromium and iron.

To make a tea, cover two teaspoons of black cohosh root with two cups of water in a pan. Bring to a boil and boil for thirty minutes. Cool and strain. Take two to three tablespoons up to six times a day, sweetened with honey, if desired.

Caution: Large doses of black cohosh can cause dizziness, nausea, and vomiting. Avoid using this herb if you are pregnant or have a history of heart disease.

See also ARTHRITIS; BRONCHITIS; CIRCULATORY DISORDERS; CRAMPS, MUSCLE; DYSMENORRHEA; EAR INFECTIONS; INFLUENZA; MACULAR DEGENERATION; PNEUMONIA; PREMENSTRUAL SYNDROME; PROSTATE PROBLEMS; SPRAINS AND STRAINS; *and* VARICOSE VEINS *in Part Two.*

Black Currant

Black currant (*Ribes nigrum*) is a tall (about six feet) deciduous bush also called quinsy berry because it is used to treat an inflammatory condition of the tonsils called quinsy. The black currant plant produces very sweet blue-black berries. In fact, its berries are popular ingredients in jams, jellies, and pies. Unfortunately, the black currant is a host for the white pine blister rust that can infest and decimate pine trees. Most areas, in an attempt to save their pine trees, do not allow the sale of black currant plants.

Black currant tea has been used to treat kidney problems, rheumatic disorders, arteriosclerosis, throat ailments, and whooping cough. The Meskwaki have used a root bark tea to expel intestinal worms. The Iroquois and the Shoshone have used a poultice made from black currant bark to treat swelling.

To make a tea, pour one cup of water over two teaspoons of dried black currant leaves and steep for five minutes. Strain. Take up to one and a half cups per day, one tablespoon at a time.

See also AGING; ALZHEIMER'S DISEASE; ARTHRITIS; BED SORES; BRUISES; CANKER SORES; CATARRH; CIRCULATORY DISORDERS; COUGHS AND COLDS; DIARRHEA; GOUT; INTESTINAL WORMS; KIDNEY AND BLADDER PROBLEMS; MACULAR DEGENERATION; SPRAINS AND STRAINS; *and* WOUNDS *in Part Two.*

Black Elder

The black elder (*Sambucus nigra*) is a shrub (sometimes a small tree) that grows up to thirty feet in height. The bark, root, leaves, flowers, and fruit are all used medicinally; however, the flowers and berries are especially effective at treating respiratory conditions. The flowers also promote perspiration, so they are helpful in treating fever and colds. The Cherokee also drank an elderberry infusion to treat rheumatism. The berries make excellent jam but should only be eaten when ripe and at least lightly cooked. To do otherwise will cause diarrhea and vomiting.

To make a tea from elderberries, pour one cup of boiling water over two tablespoons of berries. Let steep for thirty minutes. To make a tea from the black elder flowers, pour one cup of boiling water over two tablespoons of elder flowers. Take up to two hot cups of this tea a day.

See also AGING; BRONCHITIS; CATARRH; COUGHS AND COLDS; PLEURISY; PNEUMONIA; SINUSITIS; SORE THROAT; THRUSH; *and* TONSILLITIS *in Part Two.*

Black Haw

Often called American sloe or stagbush, black haw (*Viburnum prunifolium*) is a deciduous shrub or tree that can grow to about fifteen feet tall. The root and the bark of the trunk are often used as decoctions to treat dysmenorrhea (menstrual cramps). In fact, several tribes, including the Delaware, have used black haw to strengthen female reproductive organs, and many tribes have used black haw tea to prevent miscarriage. Black haw contains a chemical called scopoletin, which has been known to relax the uterus. This herb also contains salicin, which is related to aspirin and works as a pain reliever. Black haw has also been used to treat chills and fever, diarrhea and other intestinal problems, heart palpitations, and stomach problems.

To make a tea from black haw, place one tablespoon of the dried bark or root bark in a pan, cover with one cup of water, and bring to a boil. Boil for ten minutes, cool, and strain. You may want to sweeten with honey. Take half a cup at a time, up to four times a day.

Caution: Avoid using this herb if you are pregnant.

See also DYSMENORRHEA *and* PREMENSTRUAL SYNDROME *in Part Two.*

Blackberry

The blackberry (*Rubus villosus*) is a trailing perennial that grows wild almost everywhere in the United States. Blackberry goes by many names, including dewberry and brambleberry.

The Kiowa-Apache, Cherokee, Chippewa, Ojibwa, Menominee, Delaware, and Iroquois have all used a decoction made from either the blackberry roots (fresh or dried) or blackberry leaves to treat diarrhea. The Chippewa have also treated lung problems with a tea made from the roots. The Cherokee found that this root makes an effective topical wash to relieve the discomfort of hemorrhoids.

To make a tea, pour one cup of boiling water over three or four teaspoons of dried blackberry leaves. Let steep for thirty minutes and strain. Take one to two tablespoons at a time, up to one cup per day. If using the roots, place one teaspoon of the root in a pan and cover with one cup of water. Bring to a boil and boil for thirty minutes. Remove from the heat, cool, and strain. Take one to two cups per day, half a cup at a time.

See also CATARRH; DIARRHEA; FATIGUE; *and* HEMORRHOIDS *in Part Two.*

Blue Cohosh

Blue cohosh (*Caulophyllum thalictroides*) is a leafy, perennial herb that grows one to three feet in height. This herb is also called papoose root and squaw-root, which gives a good indication of its use. The Cherokee knew that the plant promotes childbirth and have used it to relieve uterine inflammation such as occurs during menstruation. The Menominee have used a root decoction to minimize heavy bleeding during menstruation, and the Chippewa have used it as a contraceptive.

Blue cohosh also has been used by the Chippewa to treat lung problems and indigestion; by the Iroquois to treat rheumatism, gallstones, and fever, and as a general tonic; by the Omaha to battle fever; and by the Cherokee to treat "fits and hysterics" and toothache. In addition to containing healing phytochemicals, blue cohosh is very high in iron, manganese, phosphorus, and selenium, and high in niacin, riboflavin, and thiamin.

To make a tea, pour two cups of boiling water over one teaspoon of granulated root in a container. Cover the container and steep for thirty minutes. Take up to one cup per day, a tablespoon at a time.

Caution: Blue cohosh can cause contact dermatitis and may irritate mucous membranes. Avoid if you have a history of heart problems. Avoid if you are pregnant because blue cohosh has an estrogenic effect. A recent article published in the *Journal of Pediatrics* told of a newborn infant who suffered congestive heart failure and shock because the mother ingested blue cohosh during labor, apparently in an attempt to promote uterine contractions. The baby eventually recovered, but he was critically ill for several weeks. Although several groups of Native Americans use blue cohosh to promote delivery, I do not recommend it for this, as it could be dangerous. If you wish to use blue cohosh during delivery, do so only under the care of a well-trained health-care provider.

See also INDIGESTION *and* INTESTINAL WORMS *in Part Two.*

Blue Flag

Blue flag (*Iris versicolor*) is a perennial herb that can grow up to three feet in height. Also known as poison flag, liver lily, and fleur-de-lis, the iris flowers from this plant are a beautiful blue. Blue flag is considered helpful in treating liver problems and has been used for this purpose by the Hudson Bay Cree and the Delaware. Blue flag also is used to treat indigestion and heartburn, gallbladder problems, and sinus problems. Topically, an infusion of blue flag leaves can be used to treat skin sores and burns.

To make a tea, pour two cups of boiling water over one teaspoon of blue flag root. Take up to one cup per day, one or two tablespoons at a time.

Caution: Blue flag may cause contact dermatitis in sensitive individuals. Use with care.

See also LIVER PROBLEMS *in Part Two.*

Blue Vervain

Also called Indian hyssop, Simpler's joy, and wild hyssop, blue vervain (*Verbena hastata*) is a perennial herb native to the northern United States and Canada. The plant grows up to five feet in height and produces blue flowers—hence its name. Blue vervain is probably best known as an effective treatment for coughs, colds, and other respiratory conditions and fever; but it is also an effective natural tranquilizer. This herb has also been used by Native Americans as a treatment for circulatory problems, headache, insomnia, and hepatitis. The Iroquois made a root decoction from blue vervain and used it to treat worms. The Menominee have used the roots in a tea to clear cloudy urine. The Teton Dakota treated stomachache with a decoction made from the leaves. In fact, the dried leaves, flowers, and the whole plant have also been used to treat a wide variety of digestive disorders. Blue vervain works in much the same way as aspirin, although it is not chemically the same.

To make a tea, pour two cups of boiling water over two teaspoons of dried blue vervain leaves. Steep for fifteen to twenty minutes, then strain. Blue vervain is bitter, so you may want to sweeten with honey. Take up to two cups a day, a tablespoon or two at a time.

Caution: Avoid blue vervain if you have a history of heart disease or if you are pregnant.

See also ARTHRITIS; ASTHMA; CATARRH; COUGHS AND COLDS; DYSMENORRHEA; FATIGUE; INTESTINAL WORMS; LIVER PROBLEMS; NERVOUSNESS; SORE THROAT; TONSILLITIS; *and* WOUNDS *in Part Two.*

Boneset

Boneset (*Eupatorium perfoliatum*) is a perennial herb that grows to about five feet in height and is indigenous to the United States. Also called ague weed and feverwort, boneset has been widely used by Native Americans for a number of ailments. The Iroquois, Mohegan, Menominee, Delaware, and Cherokee have all used boneset to treat colds and fever. The Alabama relieved stomachache with boneset tea. This herb was also used by several tribes, including the Cherokee, as a laxative.

According to herbalist Michael Weiner, there are at least thirty species of boneset in the United States. Weiner says that boneset got its name not because of any ability to mend broken bones, but because it is effective against breakbone fever (conventionally termed *dengue*), a mosquito-transmitted viral infection marked by chills, fever, headache, and muscle and bone pain. Dengue fever is common in subtropical and tropical areas. It is the leading cause of childhood mortality in several Asian countries.

Boneset is very high in magnesium and high in calcium, niacin, and phosphorus. It also contains beneficial phytochemicals, including quercetin.

To make a tea, pour one cup of boiling water over one teaspoon of dried boneset. Steep for ten to fifteen minutes and strain. Add honey to sweeten. Take one to two tablespoons up to five times a day.

Caution: Do not use fresh boneset leaves. Use dried leaves instead, since drying eliminates some of the potentially toxic chemicals present in the leaves. Avoid taking boneset if you are pregnant.

See also CATARRH; CONSTIPATION; COUGHS AND COLDS; *and* PLEURISY *in Part Two.*

Burdock

Eaten around the world as a tasty vegetable, the root of burdock (*Arctium* sp.) has long been used to treat gastrointestinal ailments (including stomach pains) and to relieve respiratory problems such as pleurisy and coughs. Also known as cocklebur and bardana, burdock has been used by the Delaware and Cherokee to treat rheumatism and by the Cherokee and Iroquois to purify the blood and aid circulation. It may be valuable as an aid to circulation because of its antioxidant and anti-inflammatory activity. Pulverized burdock leaves placed directly on the skin are helpful in treating skin sores and skin ulcers. This may be because burdock contains certain chemicals that kill bacteria and fungi. Burdock also is very high in chromium, iron, magnesium, and thiamin and high in phosphorus, potassium, vitamin A, and zinc.

To make a tea, place one teaspoon of burdock root in two cups of cold water. Bring to a boil and boil for thirty minutes. Cool and strain. Take up to two cups per day, a few tablespoons at a time.

Caution: Avoid if you are pregnant.

See also ACNE; AGING; BEDSORES; CIRCULATORY DISORDERS; COLD SORES; ECZEMA; GOUT; LIVER PROBLEMS; MONONUCLEOSIS; PSORIASIS; *and* SKIN RASH *in Part Two.*

Canadian Fleabane

Canadian fleabane (*Erigeron canadensis*) is an annual (sometimes biennial) herb that grows up to three feet in height. Indigenous to North America, it is also called coltstail, horseweed, and fleawort. Native Americans have used many types of fleabane to treat diarrhea, hemorrhoids, menstrual irregularities, and intestinal worm infestations. The Navajo have used fleabane in a lotion as a treatment for body pain and headaches.

To make a tea from fleabane, pour one cup of water over one teaspoon of the leaves. Let steep for thirty minutes. Strain. Take up to two cups a day, half a cup at a time.

See also BRONCHITIS; CANCEROUS TUMORS; CATARRH; COLITIS; DIARRHEA; INTESTINAL WORMS; SORE THROAT; *and* TONSILLITIS *in Part Two.*

Cascara Sagrada

Perhaps no plant is better known for its ability to relieve constipation than cascara sagrada (*Rhamnus purshiana*). In fact, cascara has been listed in the *United States Pharmacopoeia* as a cure for constipation since 1890. It is still widely used today as a component in many over-the-counter laxatives.

Also called chittem bark and sacred bark (*cascara sagrada* is Spanish for "sacred bark"), cascara comes from a deciduous tree indigenous to western North America, cascara buckthorn. Historically, it has been widely used by Native American tribes, including the Warm Spring, the Paiute, and the Pomo of northern California; the Thompson Indians of British Columbia; and the Nisqually. Pacific Northwest cascara is high in cobalt and vitamin A.

To make a tea from cascara sagrada, pour two cups of boiling water over one teaspoon of the dried bark. Boil for thirty minutes and strain before drinking. It is important to use bark that has aged at least a year (fresh bark is nauseating). Cascara is very bitter, so you may want to sweeten the tea with honey. Take one tablespoon at a time, up to two cups per day.

Caution: Recent reports indicate that cascara can decrease the absorption of certain drugs, so be sure to advise your physician if you are using cascara and also taking other drugs.

See also ARTHRITIS *and* CONSTIPATION *in Part Two.*

Catnip

Catnip (*Nepeta cataria*) is a perennial herb, loved by cats, that is also known as catmint. A member of the mint family, catnip grows to about three feet in height.

Several tribes have used catnip to treat coughs, colds, pneumonia, sore throats, fevers, and colic. It has sedative and diuretic properties and is also used to relieve upset stomach and flatulence. The Mohegan relieved infant colic with a tea made from the leaves of catnip. It is very high in chromium, iron, manganese, potassium, and selenium; and is high in cobalt.

To make a tea from catnip, pour one cup of boiling water over two teaspoons of catnip leaves. Steep for ten to fifteen minutes and then strain. Take up to two cups of the warm tea per day.

See also DIARRHEA; FATIGUE; FLATULENCE; HANGOVER; HEADACHE; HEARTBURN; INDIGESTION; INSOMNIA; INTESTINAL WORMS; NAUSEA AND VOMITING; *and* PNEUMONIA *in Part Two.*

Cayenne

Cayenne (*Capsicum annuum frutescens*), also called chili pepper, is a perennial plant that grows to about three feet in height. Although cayenne peppers are popular as spicy additions to many dishes, they are also used as general stimulants. When used topically, cayenne is effective at increasing blood flow to the skin, so it is helpful in treating those afflicted with arthritis or rheumatism. In fact, the Apache, Hopi, Navajo, Pueblo, and other Southwestern tribes rubbed powdered cayenne onto their arthritic joints to help block pain and reduce swelling.

To make a tea from cayenne, pour one cup of boiling water over one teaspoon of dried cayenne pepper. Let steep for twenty minutes and strain. Take one tablespoon at a time, one to two cups a day.

Caution: Cayenne can cause contact dermatitis and even blisters, so use with caution when using topically.

See also AGING; ARTHRITIS; CATARRH; CIRCULATORY DISORDERS; CONSTIPATION; DIARRHEA; HAIR LOSS; INFLUENZA; MONONUCLEOSIS; SORE THROAT; *and* TONSILLITIS *in Part Two.*

Chamomile

Chamomile (*Matricaria chamomilla*) is an annual herb indigenous to Europe that has been naturalized in North America. The plant grows to about three feet in height and has daisylike flowers. The entire plant, especially the flowers, has been used to treat a variety of ailments ranging from the common cold (and related conditions) to liver disorders, wounds and burns, insomnia, and gastrointestinal problems, including indigestion. Chamomile makes an effective poultice to heal wounds and relieve inflammation.

To make a chamomile tea, pour one cup of boiling water over two tablespoons of fresh or dried chamomile flowers. Cover and let stand for ten to fifteen minutes. Take up to two cups per day, as needed.

Caution: Individuals with ragweed allergies may be sensitive to chamomile.

See also ARTHRITIS; BRONCHITIS; CONJUNCTIVITIS; COUGHS AND COLDS; DYSMENORRHEA; FLATULENCE; HEADACHE; HEARTBURN; INDIGESTION; INFLUENZA; INSOMNIA; NAUSEA AND VOMITING; NERVOUSNESS; PLEURISY; PNEUMONIA; SUNBURN; *and* WOUNDS *in Part Two.*

Chaparral

Chaparral (*Larrea divaricata; L. tridentata*) is a perennial bush that grows in the American Southwest. Chaparral is also called creosote bush and greasewood because it has a very distinctive and extremely unpleasant smell. Chaparral has antimicrobial, anticancer, and antioxidant properties. Chaparral reportedly is effective at treating a variety of conditions, including arthritis, rheumatism, bruises, diarrhea, stomach problems, influenza, venereal disease, and even cancer. The Maricopa, Papago, and Pimas treated bruises and rheumatism by applying poultices made by boiling the leaves and branches. Topically, chaparral has been used to treat toothache and may be effective at preventing cavities. Chaparral contains beneficial flavonoids and is high in calcium, potassium, selenium, thiamin, vitamin A, and vitamin C.

To make a tea, pour one cup of boiling water over one teaspoon of the dried chaparral leaves, steep for ten to fifteen minutes, and strain. You may want to sweeten it with honey. Take one teaspoon as needed.

Caution: Extended use may be toxic to the liver.

See also HANGOVER; HEARTBURN; LIVER PROBLEMS; NAUSEA AND VOMITING; STEATORRHEA; *and* TOOTHACHE *in Part Two.*

NATIVE
AMERICAN
HERBS

35

Chicory

The root of the chicory (*Cichorium intybus*) is a common coffee substitute that has a long history of use by Native Americans. Also known as garden chicory, endive, and succory, chicory leaves can be cooked and eaten like spinach. Chicory has been used by various tribes as a liver purifier and as an aid for upset stomachs. The Cherokee found it useful as a nerve tonic. When applied topically, the bruised leaves can help relieve swelling and inflammation.

To make a chicory tea, place one teaspoon of chicory root in one cup of cold water. Bring to a boil, remove from heat, and strain. Take up to two cups a day, a tablespoon at a time.

See also LIVER PROBLEMS *in Part Two.*

Coltsfoot

Coltsfoot (*Tussilago farfara*) is a low-growing perennial herb also called British tobacco and horsehoof. Coltsfoot contains a phytochemical known as tussilagone, a potent cardiovascular and respiratory stimulant. The leaves (either dried or fresh) from this herb have been used to treat respiratory conditions including colds, coughs, bronchitis, asthma, whooping cough, tuberculosis, and influenza, as well as sinus problems and sore throats. The Lummi Indians also have used coltsfoot as an emetic.

Coltsfoot leaves are effective when used topically in a compress to treat swelling, as a poultice to treat rheumatism, or in a decoction to relieve itching.

To make a tea from coltsfoot, pour one cup of boiling water over one to two teaspoons of coltsfoot leaves. Let steep for thirty minutes and strain. Take up to one cup per day, a tablespoon at a time.

Caution: Use of this herb is controversial because it contains certain alkaloids that may be toxic to the liver or carcinogenic in nature. Use this herb cautiously and avoid entirely if you are pregnant.

See also ASTHMA; BRONCHITIS; CATARRH; CHICKENPOX; COUGHS AND

COLDS; LARYNGITIS; PLEURISY; PNEUMONIA; SORE THROAT; THRUSH; and
TUBERCULOSIS in Part Two.

Comfrey

Comfrey (*Symphytum officinale*) is a perennial herb that grows from one to
four feet in height. It has long been used in the United States to treat coughs,
gastrointestinal problems, bruises, strains, and other injuries. It is now
generally believed that comfrey should not be taken internally because it
contains certain alkaloids that have carcinogenic effects and are toxic to
the liver. Comfrey does, however, contain chemicals that can help heal
cuts, burns, and other skin problems. So, when used topically in poultices,
it is a safe and effective treatment for wounds, burns, bruises, boils, and
swellings.

To make an infusion for topical use, place two teaspoons of comfrey root in
a pan, cover with one cup of boiling water, steep thirty minutes, cool, and
strain. Use as a wash for skin conditions.

See also BITES AND STINGS, INSECTS; CATARRH; ECZEMA; PSORIASIS; SKIN
RASH; SORE THROAT; and THRUSH in Part Two.

Coneflower

Not to be confused with the purple coneflower (echinacea), coneflower (*Rudbeckia laciniata*) is a perennial herb that grows up to seven feet in height and
has yellow flowers. Also called goldenglow, coneflower is soothing to the
digestive organs, as the Chippewa discovered. They have used a tea made
from coneflower to treat indigestion. When applied topically in a poultice,
coneflower is effective at treating burns.

To make a tea, pour one cup of boiling water over one teaspoon of coneflower root, steep for thirty minutes, and then strain. Take as needed.

See also BURNS; INDIGESTION; and SUNBURN in Part Two.

Coriander

Coriander (*Coriandrum sativum*), also called cilantro, is an annual herb that grows to about three feet in height. Many of us are familiar with cilantro leaves, which are widely used in Mexican cooking.

Coriander is a digestive aid and has the ability to break up intestinal gas, so it is used to treat flatulence and other digestive complaints. Coriander contains chemicals that kill bacteria and some fungi, so it has been used to treat a wide variety of diseases including dysentery, fever, coughs and colds, and bladder disorders. Recent research indicates that coriander also has insulin-like activity, so it may be helpful in treating diabetes.

To make a tea from coriander, pour one cup of boiling water over two teaspoons of dried coriander seeds and steep for five minutes. Strain and drink up to two cups a day.

See also DIABETES *and* HEARTBURN *in Part Two.*

Corn Silk

Corn silk refers to the soft, fine, yellow threads found at the tip of an ear of corn (*Zea mays*). Corn silk has been used to soothe irritated tissues and also functions as a diuretic, which is why it is beneficial in treating premenstrual syndrome. It is a mild stimulant and is also useful in treating bladder problems.

To make a tea, pour half a cup of boiling water over one teaspoon of fresh or dried corn silk. Allow to steep for five minutes and then strain. Take every few hours, a tablespoon at a time, up to two cups a day.

See also PREMENSTRUAL SYNDROME *in Part Two.*

Couch Grass

Couch grass (*Elymus repens; Agropyron repens*) is a perennial grass that many consider a weed. Also called quack grass, this herb is high in nutritive value. The rhizome (the rootstalk) of the couch grass has been used to treat urinary tract infections and inflammation, as well as colds, fevers, and bronchitis. Native Americans have also used various types of couch grass as food sources, both for themselves and for their horses and sheep.

To make a tea from couch grass, pour one cup of water over one teaspoon of the couch grass rhizome. Let steep for ten minutes and strain. Take half a cup four or five times daily.

See also PROSTATE PROBLEMS *in Part Two.*

Crampbark

Crampbark (*Viburnum opulus*) is a tall (up to fifteen feet high) deciduous shrub that is also called high-bush cranberry, squaw bush, and European cranberry bush. The inner bark of the crampbark makes an effective relaxant, able to relieve cramps and spasms. Many tribes, including the Iroquois, Shuswap, and Ojibwa have used crampbark berries for food. The Iroquois have also used the berries to treat liver and blood conditions. The Micmac, Penobscot, and Malecite Indians have used the bark to treat swollen glands and related conditions such as mumps.

Crampbark is very high in calcium, chromium, and cobalt. It also contains high levels of several minerals including iron, magnesium, and silicon.

This herb was listed in the *United States Pharmacopoeia* between 1894 and 1916 as a sedative and antispasmodic; it is particularly effective at relieving muscle spasms from back pain and menstrual pain.

To make a crampbark tea, cover one teaspoonful of the bark with one cup of water in a pan. Boil for thirty minutes. Cool and strain. Take up to one cup per day.

See also DYSMENORRHEA *and* PREMENSTRUAL SYNDROME *in Part Two.*

Dandelion

Dandelion (*Taraxacum officinale*) is a perennial herb, found almost everywhere. Most of us think of dandelions as weeds to be eliminated from our lawns. But dandelion, also called lion's tooth and wild endive, has long been used as a laxative, diuretic, tonic, and as an aid for liver problems, including jaundice. There is also some evidence that dandelion can aid in weight loss. Dandelion greens are rich sources of iron, potassium, and vitamin A and good sources of calcium, fiber, and vitamin C.

In addition to the above uses, Native Americans have used dandelion to treat skin problems such as acne, eczema, and hives. The Pillager-Ojibwa made a dandelion root tea as treatment for heartburn, while the Cherokee used such a tea to calm the nerves. The Iroquois used dandelion for a wide range of conditions, including anemia, constipation, pain, and water retention. Many tribes chewed the dried sap like chewing gum and even roasted the root, using it like coffee.

To make a dandelion tea, pour two cups of boiling water over two tablespoons of pesticide-free dandelion leaves. Steep for fifteen minutes. Drink up to two cups per day, a tablespoon at a time. To make a tea from the roots, boil one teaspoon of dandelion root in about three cups of water for thirty minutes. Remove from the heat, and cool. Drink up to two cups per day, one tablespoon at a time.

See also ACNE; CONSTIPATION; DIABETES; FLATULENCE; GOUT; HEARTBURN; HEMORRHOIDS; LIVER PROBLEMS; *and* OBESITY *in Part Two.*

Devil's Claw

Devil's claw (*Harpagophytum procumbens*) is a perennial herb. Also called grapple plant, this herb contains anti-inflammatory components, so it is used to treat conditions marked by inflammation, such as arthritis and rheumatism. The tubular secondary roots are also used to treat pain, dyspepsia, loss of appetite, and liver and gallbladder complaints. Devil's claw is very high in cobalt, iron, and magnesium, and is high in manganese, niacin, sodium, and zinc.

To make a tea from devil's claw, pour one cup of water over one teaspoon of devil's claw roots. Soak overnight. Strain. Take half a cup at a time, up to three times a day.

Caution: Devil's claw stimulates secretion of gastric juices, so it should be avoided by anyone suffering from a stomach ulcer. It may also stimulate uterine muscles, so avoid during pregnancy.

See also ARTHRITIS; CANCEROUS TUMORS; *and* LIVER PROBLEMS *in Part Two.*

Echinacea

Echinacea (*Echinacea angustifolia; E. purpurea*), also called purple coneflower, is widely used today as a remedy for colds, coughs, and other respiratory problems and is one of the biggest-selling herbs. But the Kiowa, Cheyenne, Lakota, Arapaho, Crow, and other tribes have known of echinacea's power for centuries. Echinacea has long been used to treat fevers, bites and stings, toothaches, burns, and other painful conditions. Indians of the Upper Missouri River area treated bites (including snakebites) and stings with the macerated root. The Blackfoot chewed the root to help alleviate toothache, while several tribes used the juice from the plant to treat burns, wounds, ulcers, and other skin conditions. Echinacea has the ability to work with your immune system, strengthening it to not only prevent but also fight infections. Echinacea is very high in zinc and high in chromium, iron, manganese, niacin, riboflavin, selenium, and vitamin C.

To make a tea from echinacea, pour one cup of boiling water over one teaspoon of the granulated root. Let steep for thirty minutes and strain. Take one tablespoon of the tea up to six times per day.

See also ABSCESS; ACNE; ASTHMA; BEDSORES; BOILS; BRONCHITIS;

Burns; Cancerous Tumors; Candidiasis; Canker Sores; Catarrh; Cold Sores; Coughs and Colds; Ear Infections; Eczema; Fatigue; Indigestion; Intestinal Worms; Liver Problems; Malaise; Measles; Mononucleosis; Pleurisy; Ringworm; Sinusitis; Skin Rash; Sore Throat; Sunburn; Tonsillitis; *and* Wounds *in Part Two.*

Elecampane

Elecampane (*Inula helenium*) is a perennial herb that grows up to six feet in height. Also called elf dock and scabwort, elecampane root is best known for its ability to soothe coughing. The Algonquin, Cherokee, Delaware, Iroquois, and others have used this herb to treat various respiratory problems, including tuberculosis, asthma, and the common cold. Scientists have now verified that elecampane exhibits significant activity against *Mycobacterium tuberculosis*, the bacterium that causes tuberculosis.

Elecampane has also been used to improve digestion. In fact, the Delaware made a tonic from the root to strengthen the digestive organs. This herb is very high in magnesium, thiamin, and zinc and high in calcium and niacin.

To make a tea, cover one teaspoon of the root with two cups of water in a pan. Bring to a boil and boil for thirty minutes. Remove from heat, cover, and steep until cool. Strain. Sweeten with honey and take up to two cups a day, a tablespoon or so at a time.

Caution: Avoid this herb if you are pregnant.

See also Asthma; Bronchitis; Coughs and Colds; Croup; Dysmenorrhea; Intestinal Worms; Liver Problems; *and* Tuberculosis *in Part Two.*

Evening Primrose

Evening primrose (*Oenothera biennis*) is an annual or biennial herb that can grow up to seven feet in height. Also called king's cure-all, fever plant, and scurvish, this herb has been used as both a tea and a topical wash by the Iroquois to treat hemorrhoids. Evening primrose is also an effective remedy for coughs and colds, depression, and digestive problems. In poultices, it has been used to treat bruises and boils as well as skin rashes and other skin irritations.

Evening primrose produces a seed that is rich in oils containing gamma-linolenic acid (GLA). It is believed that GLA can improve the body's production of hormonelike compounds that can reduce inflammation and increase blood flow.

To make a tea, pour one cup of boiling water over one teaspoon of the herb. Take up to one cup a day, a tablespoon at a time.

See also BEDSORES; HEMORRHOIDS; PREMENSTRUAL SYNDROME; *and* SKIN RASH *in Part Two.*

Feverfew

Also called featherfew, feverfew (*Tanacetum parthenium*) is an aromatic perennial that grows nearly three feet in height and is related to the chamomile plant. This herb is used primarily to treat arthritis, headaches, and allergies, but it can also improve digestion. When used topically, it is an effective antiseptic.

Many people use feverfew to treat migraine headaches. Scientists have found that taking feverfew can reduce the number and severity of migraine attacks, as well as the degree of vomiting that often accompanies a migraine.

Feverfew is very high in niacin and contains high amounts of chromium, magnesium, manganese, phosphorus, potassium, selenium, and thiamin.

To make a tea, pour one cup of boiling water over one teaspoon of feverfew leaves, steep for ten minutes, and strain. Add honey, as feverfew is bitter. Take one tablespoon at a time throughout the day, up to two cups per day.

Caution: Avoid feverfew if you are taking blood-thinning drugs.

See also ARTHRITIS; CATARRH; DYSMENORRHEA; HEADACHE; INTESTINAL WORMS; *and* WOUNDS *in Part Two.*

Fringe Tree

The fringe tree (*Chionanthus virginicus*), also called old-man's-beard, grows up to twenty-five feet in height and blooms in fragrant white flowers in late spring. The bark of the fringe tree is used as a diuretic to increase the expulsion of urine. It also functions as a gentle purgative and can reduce fevers and strengthen the entire body. It has been used to treat dyspepsia, kidney and liver problems, and prostate problems. The Choctaw have used a bark decoction topically to treat cuts, bruises, and infected sores.

To make a tea, cover one teaspoon of the bark with one cup of boiling water in a pan. Bring to a boil and boil for five to ten minutes. Take up to one cup per day.

See also PROSTATE PROBLEMS *in Part Two.*

Ginger

The root of the ginger (*Zingiberis rhizoma*) is a popular ingredient in Chinese dishes because of the tangy taste it imparts. It has been used in Asian medicine for nearly 3,000 years. Although it is native to tropical Asia, as with many herbs, it was brought to North America long ago and gradually worked its way into Native American use.

Ginger can improve appetite, helps expel flatulence, increases perspiration, stimulates saliva secretion, and also acts as a stimulant. Ginger is effective at relieving a number of conditions, including coughs and colds, influenza, motion sickness, pleurisy, and digestive problems. Adding ginger to almost any medicinal mixture can improve the effect of the main ingredient. Ginger root is very high in manganese and silicon and high in magnesium and potassium.

To make a tea, pour one cup of boiling water over one to two slices of fresh ginger root or two teaspoons of the grated root. Steep for ten to fifteen minutes, strain, and sweeten with honey if desired.

See also ACNE; AGING; BITES AND STINGS, INSECTS; BOILS; BRONCHITIS; CANCEROUS TUMORS; CIRCULATORY DISORDERS; CONSTIPATION; COUGHS

AND COLDS; DIARRHEA; EAR INFECTIONS; FLATULENCE; HEARTBURN; INDI-
GESTION; INFLUENZA; NAUSEA AND VOMITING; NERVOUSNESS; PLEURISY;
SINUSITIS; *and* STRESS *in Part Two.*

Ginkgo Biloba

Ginkgo biloba is a tree (also called the maidenhair tree) that is considered the
longest-surviving tree species. The Chinese have used ginkgo for thousands of
years. As was the case with other herbs, immigrants introduced ginkgo to North
America, where it has slowly but surely gained a foothold in herbal medicine.

Ginkgo improves circulation, thereby improving the delivery of necessary
nutrients and life-giving oxygen to every cell, including those of the brain.
This is why ginkgo is so widely touted as a memory aid and fatigue fighter.
Ginkgo has also been shown to enhance energy and reduce depression. In
addition to beneficial phytochemicals, including ginkgolic acid, ginkgo is
very high in chromium and niacin and high in calcium, phosphorus, selenium, and zinc.

To make a tea, pour two cups of boiling water over two teaspoons of *Ginkgo
biloba* leaves. Steep for thirty minutes. Strain and cool. Take one-quarter to
half a cup per day.

Caution: Avoid this herb if you are taking warfarin, a blood thinner, since
ginkgo inhibits the action of platelet activity factor (PAF), a key component of
the blood's clotting mechanism.

See also ACNE; AGING; ALZHEIMER'S DISEASE; BITES AND STINGS, INSECT;
BOILS; CHRONIC FATIGUE SYNDROME; CIRCULATORY DISORDERS; COUGHS
AND COLDS; EAR INFECTION; FATIGUE; MACULAR DEGENERATION; PLEURISY;
SINUSITIS; SPRAINS AND STRAINS; *and* VARICOSE VEINS *in Part Two.*

Ginseng

American ginseng (*Panax quinquefolium* or *P. quinquefolius*) is a perennial
herb used as a general tonic and a stimulant, as well as to fight fatigue, soothe

irritated mucous membranes, and strengthen the stomach. Although recent research has substantiated ginseng's beneficial effects, Native Americans have known about it for centuries. The Delaware, Algonquin, Iroquois, Mohegan, Cherokee, Menominee, and others have long used ginseng root as a tonic. The root juice was also used on wounds and sores by the Alabama Creek, while the Iroquois have used root infusions as eyedrops and eardrops.

There are currently a number of ginseng products on the market promoted as "fatigue fighters." To see if ginseng really could have an effect on fatigue and endurance, scientists took two groups of mice, giving one group ginseng supplements and the other a harmless (and useless) placebo. They then subjected both groups of mice to a swimming endurance test. The mice taking ginseng were able to swim significantly longer before reaching exhaustion than the mice not receiving ginseng.

Researchers around the world have been testing ginseng's effectiveness against everything from cancer to ulcers. Compounds isolated from ginseng have been found to be effective at inhibiting human ovarian cancer cell growth, improving immunity, reducing cholesterol, reducing blood sugar levels in diabetics, protecting the liver, and enhancing appetite.

To make a ginseng tea, cover one teaspoon of dried ginseng root with two cups of water in a pan. Bring to a boil; reduce heat and simmer for ten minutes. Cool and strain. Take up to two cups a day.

See also ACNE; AGING; ASTHMA; CANCEROUS TUMORS; CHRONIC FATIGUE SYNDROME; CIRCULATORY DISORDERS; CRAMPS, MUSCLE; DIABETES; FATIGUE; INTESTINAL WORMS; MONONUCLEOSIS; SINUSITIS; *and* SPRAINS AND STRAINS *in Part Two.*

Goldenrod

Goldenrod (*Solidago* sp.) is a perennial herb that grows up to four feet in height. Also called blue mountain tea, goldenrod is especially beneficial in treating coughs, colds, and sore throats because it can reduce nasal secretions. The leaves of this plant have also been used to decrease flatulence, promote perspiration, and increase urine secretion.

The Chippewa chewed the dried roots to relieve sore throats, while the Zuni chewed the crushed blossoms for the same reason. The Chippewa also drank a decoction made from the roots to treat lung trouble. Because goldenrod is an astringent, it was used by the Thompson Indians, Okanagan Indians, and others to treat diarrhea.

Poultices made from the flowers have been used to treat burns and skin ulcers. The Chippewa applied warm compresses made by boiling the stalk or the root to treat sprains or strained muscles.

To make a tea, pour one cup of boiling water over one teaspoon of goldenrod leaves. Take up to half a cup at a time, up to two cups a day.

See also BURNS; CATARRH; COUGHS AND COLDS; GOUT; HEMORRHOIDS; PROSTATE PROBLEMS; SORE THROAT; SUNBURN; TONSILLITIS; TUBERCULOSIS; *and* WOUNDS *in Part Two.*

Goldenseal

Goldenseal (*Hydrastis canadensis*) is a small, perennial herb whose root is used as a general tonic, as well as to improve circulation, fight coughs and colds, and bolster general health. Goldenseal is an effective antiseptic, a gentle purgative, and a diuretic. The Iroquois drank goldenseal root infusions and decoctions to treat fevers and pneumonia, while several tribes have used goldenseal to fight tuberculosis. It has also been used to treat eye ailments, skin problems, and earaches. In probably its most interesting use, the Cherokee smeared a combination of bear fat and goldenseal root on their bodies to repel insects.

Goldenseal contains very high levels of cobalt and silicon and high amounts of iron, magnesium, manganese, vitamin C, and zinc.

To make a tea, pour two cups of boiling water over one teaspoon of the dried and powdered goldenseal root. Let steep for ten to fifteen minutes and strain. You may want to add honey or some other sweetener since goldenseal is bitter. Take one to two teaspoons at a time, up to one cup a day for no more than seven days.

Caution: Avoid goldenseal if you have high blood pressure or if you are pregnant or nursing.

See also AGING; ALLERGIES; ASTHMA; CIRCULATORY DISORDERS; COLD SORES; COUGHS AND COLDS; DIABETES; ECZEMA; HANGOVER; MALAISE; MEASLES; MONONUCLEOSIS; PNEUMONIA; PROSTATE PROBLEMS; SINUSITIS; SKIN RASH; TONSILLITIS; TOOTHACHE; TUBERCULOSIS; *and* WOUNDS *in Part Two.*

Gotu Kola

Gotu kola (*Centella asiatica*) is a low, creeping herb that has been used for centuries in India, China, and the South Pacific. Related to the carrot, gotu kola supports the integrity of collagen and skin. It can help heal minor wounds and skin irritations, help ensure blood vessel integrity, and promote circulation throughout the body, including circulation to the brain. Gotu kola contains very high levels of manganese, sodium, thiamin, and vitamin A and high amounts of calcium, magnesium, niacin, riboflavin, and zinc.

To make a tea, pour one cup of boiling water over one teaspoon of gotu kola leaves. Steep for thirty minutes and strain. Gotu kola is bitter, so add a sweetener, if desired. Take two to three tablespoons, as needed.

See also ACNE; ALZHEIMER'S DISEASE; CHRONIC FATIGUE SYNDROME; CIRCULATORY DISORDERS; FATIGUE; *and* SPRAINS AND STRAINS *in Part Two.*

Ground Ivy

Ground ivy (*Nepeta hederacea*) is a creeping perennial herb that has a mint-like odor. Also called cat's foot and cat's paw, this perennial herb has been used to improve digestion and increase urine secretion. It also appears to improve lung diseases and is a stimulant and a tonic. It has been used as an astringent and to relieve diarrhea. It can also help reduce excessive mucous membrane secretions as occur in bronchitis, colds, pneumonia, and sore throats.

To make a tea from ground ivy, pour one cup of water over one teaspoon of ground ivy leaves. Take up to one cup per day.

Caution: Large doses of ground ivy may be poisonous. If in doubt, check with a herbalogist.

See also ALLERGIES; FATIGUE; *and* PNEUMONIA *in Part Two.*

Hops

Hops (*Humulus americana* and *H. lupulus*) is probably best known as an additive that helps preserve beer, but this herb has long been used as a sedative. The fruit from this perennial vine can also help relieve pain and fever and is an effective diuretic and digestive aid. Native Americans, including the Algonquin and Mohegan (among others), have used the blossoms to treat nervousness. In addition, the Fox and Cherokee used the plant as a sedative. The Mohegan used a blossom infusion to relieve toothaches.

Hops are very high in niacin and high in manganese, phosphorus, potassium, riboflavin, selenium, and vitamin C.

To make a tea from hops, pour half a cup of boiling water over one teaspoon of hops. Steep for fifteen minutes. You may want to add honey to sweeten. Take half a cup at a time, three times a day.

Caution: Do not take hops if you suffer from depression or if you are pregnant.

See also HEARTBURN; INSOMNIA; INTESTINAL WORMS; NERVOUSNESS; *and* STRESS *in Part Two.*

HOW TO MAKE A HOPS PILLOW

Sleeping on a hops pillow can help fight insomnia. To make a pillow, gather enough dried hops to fill a pillowcase or a small cloth bag. Place the hops in a glass bowl and lightly sprinkle them with a solution made of water with a touch of glycerin (this will minimize the noise made by the dried hops). Then place the hops in the pillowcase or cloth bag and either tie it closed with a ribbon or sew it closed.

NATIVE
AMERICAN
HERBS

49

Horehound

Horehound (*Marrubium vulgare*) is an aromatic perennial herb best known as a cure for respiratory conditions. Also called hoarhound and marrubium, this herb has been used to treat liver and gallbladder complaints, dyspepsia, appetite loss, and intestinal worms.

To make a tea, pour one cup of boiling water over one teaspoon of horehound leaves. Steep for ten to fifteen minutes before straining. Adding honey or some other sweetener can improve horehound's distinctive taste. Take up to two cups of tea a day, one tablespoon at a time. To make horehound syrup, add up to a pound of sugar to two cups of the tea; heat the solution until the sugar dissolves and continue heating and stirring until the syrup thickens.

See also ASTHMA; BRONCHITIS; CANCEROUS TUMORS; COUGHS AND COLDS; GOUT; INTESTINAL WORMS; NAUSEA AND VOMITING; PNEUMONIA; *and* TUBERCULOSIS *in Part Two.*

Horseradish

Horseradish (*Armoracia lapathifolia*) is a perennial herb whose grated root is used to make a popular condiment. This herb has been used to treat kidney, bladder, and other urinary tract infections. The Cherokee have used horseradish to treat asthma, and it is also effective at relieving coughs and bronchitis. It is a stomachic; that is, it is effective at strengthening the stomach. However, horseradish root contains certain oils that have the potential to irritate stomach ulcers, so it should be avoided by those individuals suffering from ulcers. Horseradish is also considered a rubefacient, bringing blood to the skin, turning it red. Many tribes, including the Ontario Delaware and the Mohegan, have applied poultices of the leaves to treat neuralgia and toothache.

Horseradish is very high in chromium, magnesium, phosphorus, potassium, riboflavin, vitamin A, and vitamin C and high in calcium, manganese, niacin, and zinc.

To make horseradish tea, place one cup of finely grated horseradish in a glass container and pour enough vinegar on the horseradish to cover. Let stand for one week and refrigerate. To use, place one teaspoon of the solution in half a glass of water. Sweeten with honey. Take up to three times a day.

See also KIDNEY AND BLADDER PROBLEMS *and* LIVER PROBLEMS *in Part Two.*

Horsetail

Horsetail (*Equisetum arvense*), also called shave grass, is a perennial herb that grows wild all over North America. It is an effective diuretic, something many tribes, including the Blackfoot and Okanagan, have discovered. When applied topically, horsetail can stop bleeding and help heal wounds. The Okanagan have used a solution made by boiling horsetail stems to wash skin sores. They have also treated poison ivy by washing the affected areas with a mixture of pounded horsetail and water.

Horsetail contains a number of minerals, including calcium, chromium, iron, phosphorus, and selenium, and is a common source of supplemental silica. Silica promotes bone growth and collagen formation, two very important functions. Collagen is the "glue" that holds connective tissues together.

Horsetail should never be consumed in its whole, raw state, not only because the body cannot assimilate it in this form, but because it can destroy vitamin B_1 in the body. Instead, steep horsetail in hot water before drinking.

To make a tea from horsetail, pour one cup of boiling water over two teaspoons of dried horsetail. Steep for ten to fifteen minutes and strain. Take up to one cup per day throughout the day for no longer than three days at a time.

See also ACNE; AGING; GOUT; PROSTATE PROBLEMS; SPRAINS AND STRAINS; TUBERCULOSIS; *and* WOUNDS *in Part Two.*

Hyssop

Hyssop (*Hyssopus officinalis*) is a perennial shrub that grows up to about two feet in height. It has been used to treat sore throats, coughs, colds, and other respiratory problems, a fact the Cherokee have known for centuries. It is also effective at relieving digestive problems such as flatulence. Topically, it makes an effective antiseptic wash for burns and other skin disorders.

To make a tea, pour one cup of water over two teaspoons of dried hyssop. Let stand for eight hours and strain. You may want to sweeten with honey. Take up to half a cup a day, a tablespoon at a time.

To treat burns and other skin problems, place two teaspoons of dried hyssop in boiling water; steep for fifteen to twenty minutes, until cool, and strain. Soak a clean cotton cloth in the resulting solution and then place the cloth on the affected area, as needed.

See also BRUISES; BURNS; *and* LIVER PROBLEMS *in Part Two.*

Indian Root

Indian root (*Aralia racemosa*) is a bushy, aromatic perennial also known as spikenard. The rhizome and roots of this herb are used in infusions and decoctions to treat colds and coughs and other respiratory conditions. Indian root is an expectorant, so it is effective at treating conditions marked by excess phlegm, such as asthma and bronchitis. Native Americans have used Indian root topically to treat bruises, wounds, and other skin conditions.

To make a tea, pour one cup of boiling water over one to two teaspoons of powdered Indian root. Steep for thirty minutes and then strain. Take up to two cups a day, a tablespoon at a time.

See also ASTHMA; BRONCHITIS; COUGHS AND COLDS; INFLUENZA; MALAISE; SORE THROAT; *and* TONSILLITIS *in Part Two.*

Juniper

Juniper (*Juniperus communis*) is an evergreen shrub or tree that grows anywhere from three to six feet in height but in some areas may grow to thirty feet. Juniper is also known as genvier—the term from which the word "gin" was derived. Juniper berries are used in gin's production and lend gin its distinctive taste. Juniper berries are also used in cooking. Infusions of juniper berries are used to treat arthritis and digestive problems such as flatulence. They are well known for their diuretic properties and have been used for centuries to eliminate excess water from the body. The Shoshone have used a tea made from the berries to treat kidney and bladder problems; the Canadian Cree drink a tea made from the root for the same purpose. Topically, infusions of juniper berries have been used to treat eczema, psoriasis, and other skin problems.

The juniper berry contains a number of minerals, including chromium, cobalt, and zinc, and trace amounts of several vitamins, including niacin, riboflavin, and vitamin C.

To make a tea, place one teaspoon of crushed juniper berries in a pan. Cover with half a cup of water. Steep for fifteen to twenty minutes, until cool, and strain. Take up to one cup per day, a tablespoon at a time, for no more than six weeks at a time.

Caution: Excessive use can irritate and possibly damage the kidneys. Avoid this herb if you suffer from hay fever.

See also DIABETES; HEARTBURN; INTESTINAL WORMS; *and* PROSTATE PROBLEMS *in Part Two.*

Kava Kava

Kava kava (*Piper methysticum*) is a bush that grows up to about ten feet in height. It is indigenous to the South Sea islands, where it has been used in ceremonies for thousands of years. As with many other herbs, kava kava was brought to North America long ago and has gradually worked its way into Native American use.

The dried rhizome of the kava kava plant acts as a sedative, diuretic, and muscle relaxant. Because of these properties, it has been used to treat stress, anxiety, nervousness, and insomnia.

To make a kava tea, cover two teaspoons of kava kava root with two cups of water in a container. Let stand overnight. Strain. Take half a cup up to four times daily.

Caution: Avoid this herb if you are pregnant or nursing or are currently taking any medication for depression. Excessive use of this herb can cause dry and scaly skin, liver damage, high blood pressure, blood cell abnormalities, muscle weakness, dizziness, and visual impairment.

See also EAR INFECTIONS; NERVOUSNESS; PROSTATE PROBLEMS; *and* STRESS *in Part Two.*

Lady's Slipper

Lady's slipper (*Cypripedium* sp.) is a perennial herb native to North America. Also known as nerve root, a name that gives a good indication of its usage, this plant is called lady's slipper because its flowers resemblance slippers. Lady's slipper is used to relieve nervousness, headaches, spasms, and cramps. It also appears to promote perspiration and is used as a general tonic.

The Chippewa have also used this herb topically, placing the dried and then remoistened root directly onto skin inflammations and toothaches to relieve discomfort. Please note that the Chippewa use the root; to use the leaves and plant itself may cause severe contact dermatitis.

To make a tea, cover six tablespoons of ground lady's slipper root with two cups of water in a pan. Bring to a boil; cover; remove from heat and allow to steep for one hour and then strain. Take up to a cup a day, a tablespoon at a time. Drink cold or slightly warmed.

Caution: Excessive use can cause hallucinations.

See also INTESTINAL WORMS *in Part Two.*

Licorice

Licorice (*Glycyrrhiza glabra*) is a hardy perennial herb that grows between four and eight feet in height. Licorice root has been used for thousands of years to treat bronchial and other respiratory problems. Licorice is also effective at relieving ulcer pain and treating other stomach and gastrointestinal problems. In fact, the Cheyenne have treated diarrhea and upset stomach with a tea made from dried, peeled licorice roots. Licorice has anti-inflammatory properties and is believed to stimulate the body's immune system to better fight diseases caused by bacteria, viruses, and fungi. Licorice is also an effective laxative.

Licorice root contains a substance called glycyrrhizin, which is considered to be fifty times sweeter than table sugar. The Paiute, Cheyenne, and many other tribes chewed on the root for its sweetness. In addition to its glycyrrhizin, licorice is very high in magnesium and silicon and high in chromium, cobalt, iron, and niacin.

To make a tea, pour one cup of boiling water over one teaspoon of licorice root. Let steep ten to twenty-five minutes, until cool, and strain. Drink up to one cup per day for no more than five days at a time.

Caution: Licorice contains chemicals that act in the body in much the same way as aldosterone, the hormone produced by the adrenal glands. Excessive intake can lead to water retention and elevated blood pressure, so use in moderation.

See also ACNE; BOILS; BRONCHITIS; COUGHS AND COLDS; DIABETES; EAR INFECTIONS; INDIGESTION; LARYNGITIS; PLEURISY; PREMENSTRUAL SYNDROME; SINUSITIS; SORE THROAT; SPRAINS AND STRAINS; *and* TONSILLITIS *in Part Two.*

Marigold

The common marigold (*Calendula officinalis*) is an annual herb that grows one to two feet in height and has very strong-smelling flowers. Many gardeners plant marigolds in their gardens to keep bugs away from vegetables. Infusions made from marigold flowers are used to treat a number of conditions, including stomach cramps, diarrhea, ulcers, and fever. Topically, marigold is used to heal skin inflammations such as acne, wounds, and burns.

To make a marigold tea, pour half a cup of boiling water over one to two teaspoons of fresh or dried marigold flowers. Steep for five to ten minutes and strain. Take one tablespoon every hour or two, up to one cup a day.

See also ALLERGIES; ATHLETE'S FOOT; BEDSORES; BITES AND STINGS, INSECT; BOILS; CATARRH; CHICKENPOX; *and* DYSMENORRHEA *in Part Two.*

Marshmallow

Marshmallow (*Althea officinalis*) is a perennial herb that grows two to four feet in height. It grows best in marshy areas, hence its name. Also called althea, marshmallow is widely used to treat respiratory problems because it inhibits mucus, acts as an anti-inflammatory, and is an immune stimulant.

To make a tea, pour one cup of boiling water over two tablespoons of marshmallow leaves or flowers. Let steep for five to ten minutes and strain. Alternatively, place one to two tablespoons of marshmallow root, or the entire plant, into a glass container. Cover with one cup of cold water and let stand for eight hours. Strain. Take up to two cups per day, as needed. The tea may be warmed slighty after cooking.

Caution: Use marshmallow with caution if you are taking prescription drugs, since marshmallow can alter the absorption of drugs taken at the same time.

See also BITES AND STINGS, INSECT; BOILS; BRONCHITIS; CATARRH; DIARRHEA; LARYNGITIS; MEASLES; PNEUMONIA; SINUS-

ITIS; Skin Rash; Sore Throat; Sprains and Strains; Tonsillitis; *and* Wounds *in Part Two.*

Milk Thistle

Milk thistle (*Silybum marianum*) is a tall (up to five feet in height) annual plant with a milky sap and prickly leaves. The seed of the milk thistle has been used for centuries to treat liver problems. Milk thistle contains silymarin (found in the seed case), which protects the liver from toxins (such as the death cap mushroom) and can actually help regenerate and repair the liver. This herb also appears to protect the liver from damage caused by drinking alcohol. Not surprisingly, milk thistle is used to treat liver problems, including chronic liver necroses, cirrhosis, and hepatitis A and B.

To make a tea, pour one cup of boiling water over one teaspoon of the crushed, ripe seeds; steep for thirty minutes and strain. Take half a cup at a time, up to four times daily.

See also Aging; Liver Problems; *and* Premenstrual Syndrome *in Part Two.*

Mirabilis

Mirabilis (*Mirabilis multiflorum*) is also known as wild four-o'clock and Colorado four-o'clock. Native Americans have used various species of this plant, which is native to desert and other dry areas. Southwestern Indians have relied on mirabilis root to suppress appetite, treat fevers, and as a diuretic to increase urine output. It is also used to treat stomach disorders and as a cough medicine. Topically, root poultices are applied to burns. The Navajo have also used the berries as food, either stewing or roasting them.

To make a tea, place one teaspoon of the dried root in a pan and cover with two cups of water; boil until reduced to one cup; strain. Take a quarter to half a cup before meals.

See also CANCEROUS TUMORS; CHRONIC FATIGUE SYNDROME; FATIGUE; INTESTINAL WORMS; and OBESITY in Part Two.

Mullein

Mullein (*Verbascum thapsus*) is a biennial plant that grows up to six feet in height and has distinctive velvety leaves. Mullein is well known for its effectiveness in treating respiratory problems, including bronchitis and asthma, which is why some people call it lungwort. Mullein tea is soothing and can help relieve coughing; the Catawba, Delaware, and Cherokee have made a syrup from the leaves for this purpose. Mullein tea can also relieve pain, so it is helpful in treating arthritis and other painful conditions. Many tribes, including the Cherokee, have used mullein for this purpose.

The Delaware heated the leaves and applied them as a poultice to treat the pain of rheumatism, while the Cherokee treated swollen glands by applying scalded leaves. You can also use an infusion of the leaves, or the tea, topically.

To make a tea, pour one cup of boiling water over one teaspoon of dried mullein leaves or flowers; steep for five to ten minutes. You may want to add honey, since mullein is bitter. Take up to two cups per day, a tablespoon at a time.

Caution: Avoid mullein seeds, as they are poisonous.

See also ARTHRITIS; BRONCHITIS; COUGHS AND COLDS; CROUP; HEARTBURN; LARYNGITIS; MEASLES; MONONUCLEOSIS; and WOUNDS in Part Two.

Nettle

Nettle (*Urtica dioica*), or stinging nettle, is a perennial plant found almost everywhere in the world. Native Americans have used nettle to treat bronchitis and other respiratory problems, digestive problems, urinary tract problems, and diarrhea. It also has a long history of use in treating gout.

Nettle leaf contains astringent tannins and is also very high in calcium, chromium, magnesium, and zinc.

To make a tea, pour one cup of boiling water over two tablespoons of dried nettle leaves. Let steep for twenty to thirty minutes and strain. Take as needed, up to two cups a day.

Caution: Handle nettle carefully and wear gloves if you want to gather the leaves. Stinging nettle has small needlelike projections that are extremely irritating to the skin and will burn long after contact.

See also ALLERGIES; ANEMIA; ARTHRITIS; BEDSORES; BRONCHITIS; INTESTINAL WORMS; PLEURISY; *and* PROSTATE PROBLEMS *in Part Two.*

Ocotillo Bark

The ocotillo (*Fouquieria splendens*) is a spiny plant, native to the American Southwest. Although it looks like a cactus, it isn't. The ocotillo plant can grow up to thirty feet in height and lives in dry, rocky areas. Native Americans have used this plant for centuries, usually topically to treat wounds. However, it is also effective when taken internally to treat liver and other problems. The Cahuilla utilized the blossoms to make a beverage and ground the parched seeds into a flour. The Papago made a candy by drying the blossom nectar.

To make a tea, place one teaspoon of the bark in a pan and cover with two cups of water; bring to a boil and boil until the liquid has reduced to one cup. Take a tablespoon at a time, up to four times daily.

See also COLITIS; LIVER PROBLEMS; MALAISE; PREMENSTRUAL SYNDROME; PSORIASIS; STEATORRHEA; *and* VARICOSE VEINS *in Part Two.*

Oregon Grape

Oregon grape (*Mahonia aquifolia*) is an evergreen shrub native to North America. Related to the barberry, Oregon grape is also called Rocky Mountain grape and trailing mahonia. The roots of this herb have been used by several tribes as a general tonic. It is an effective diuretic, so it has been used to treat kidney problems and the water retention that can occur because of premenstrual syndrome. A tea made from the roots also has been used as an eyewash and as a wash for skin and mouth sores. Oregon grape is also a laxative, used to treat constipation.

To make a tea, place one teaspoon of granulated Oregon grape root in a pan; cover with two cups of boiling water; steep for thirty minutes; strain. Take one tablespoon at a time, up to half a cup per day.

See also ABSCESS; ACNE; ALLERGIES; ANEMIA; BOILS; CANCEROUS TUMORS; CANKER SORES; CONJUNCTIVITIS; CONSTIPATION; DIABETES; DIARRHEA; ECZEMA; HANGOVER; HEARTBURN; INDIGESTION; KIDNEY AND BLADDER PROBLEMS; LIVER PROBLEMS; NAUSEA AND VOMITING; PREMENSTRUAL SYNDROME; PSORIASIS; SKIN RASH; *and* STEATORRHEA *in Part Two.*

Osha Root

Osha root (*Ligusticum porteri*) is a perennial herb that has a long history of use by Native Americans. Also called chuchupate, osha root is very good at fighting viral infections, such as the common cold, and is a natural antibiotic. It also causes sweating and helps eliminate toxins. Osha has been widely used by numerous tribes in rituals and ceremonies.

To make a tea, place one teaspoon of osha root in a pan and cover with one cup of boiling water. Let simmer for fifteen minutes and strain. Take up to half a cup per day, a tablespoon at a time.

See also COUGHS AND COLDS; PNEUMONIA; SORE THROAT; *and* TONSILLITIS *in Part Two.*

Oxeye Daisy

Oxeye daisy (*Chrysanthemum leucanthemum*) is a perennial herb that grows from a few inches to about three feet in height. Also called white weed and golden daisy, the leaves and flowers of this plant are used to promote sweating and to treat coughs and colds and urinary disorders.

To make a tea, pour one cup of boiling water over one teaspoon of the flowering herb. Let steep for thirty minutes and strain. Take frequently (every few hours) throughout the day.

See also ALLERGIES; CATARRH; COUGHS AND COLDS; HEARTBURN; LIVER PROBLEMS; *and* WOUNDS *in Part Two.*

Parsley

Parsley (*Petroselinum crispum*) is a biennial (sometimes annual) herb that grows almost everywhere. Most of us know parsley only as a garnish, but it is an effective diuretic. In fact, the Cherokee have used parsley to treat kidney and bladder problems. Parsley contains high levels of chlorophyll, so it works as an effective breath freshener when chewed. Parsley also contains very high levels of potassium and vitamin A and high levels of calcium, magnesium, niacin, phosphorus, riboflavin, and vitamin C.

Parsley appears to be effective when used topically. Native Americans have used parsley leaves in compresses to treat insect bites and stings, as well as swollen glands.

To make a tea, pour one cup of boiling water over one tablespoon of parsley; steep for fifteen to twenty minutes and strain. Drink up to two cups a day.

See also AGING *and* KIDNEY AND BLADDER PROBLEMS *in Part Two.*

Passionflower

Passionflower (*Passiflora incarnata*) is a perennial vine that can grow twenty-five to thirty feet in length. Passionflower contains several tranquilizing chemicals, so it is often used for its sedative properties to relieve nervousness and insomnia. It can also relax smooth muscles, such as those of the uterus and the digestive tract. The Cherokee drank a root infusion to treat liver problems, while the Housma used such a tea as a blood tonic. Topically, passionflower has been used by the Cherokee to treat boils, wounds, and earache. The Cherokee also have used it as a food and a beverage.

To make a tea, pour one cup of boiling water over one to two teaspoons of dried passionflower; steep for fifteen to twenty minutes and strain. Take up to two cups a day. If you are drinking passionflower tea to cure insomnia, drink half to one cup just before bed.

See also ASTHMA; CROUP; DYSMENORRHEA; INSOMNIA; NERVOUSNESS; *and* PREMENSTRUAL SYNDROME *in Part Two.*

Pau d'Arco

Pau d'arco (*Tabebuia impetiginosa*), also called lapacho, taheebo, trumpet bush, and ipe roxo, is both the name for a tree and for medicine made from the tree's inner bark. The tree can grow up to 125 feet tall and is native to the Americas. Pau d'arco is rich in phytochemicals called quinones. One such quinone, lapachol, is considered one of the most important antibacterial and antitumor agents around. It also has anti-inflammatory properties. Pau d'arco has been used to treat cancer, candidiasis, colds, diabetes, fever, flu, infections, malaria, sexually transmitted diseases, and wounds.

In addition to quinones and other beneficial phytochemicals, pau d'arco is also very high in calcium and cobalt and high in silicon.

To make a tea, place one teaspoon of pau d'arco bark in a glass container and cover with one cup of cold water; let soak overnight. Take half a cup up to three times a day.

See also ATHLETE'S FOOT; CANDIDIASIS; MEASLES; MONONUCLEOSIS; RINGWORM; SINUSITIS; *and* THRUSH *in Part Two.*

Pearly Everlasting

Pearly everlasting (*Anaphalis margaritacea*) is a perennial herb that grows to about two feet in height. Also called Indian posy, pearly everlasting is an effective expectorant. In fact, Native Americans have long used the herb to treat lung problems. It has also been used to relieve diarrhea and intestinal problems, including hemorrhage. The Algonquin have used pearly everlasting tea to strengthen female reproductive organs.

To make a tea, pour one cup of boiling water over one teaspoon of pearly everlasting flowers and leaves; steep for fifteen to twenty minutes and strain. Take up to two cups a day, a tablespoon at a time.

See also ALLERGIES *and* BRONCHITIS *in Part Two.*

Peppermint

Peppermint (*Mentha piperita*) is a perennial herb that grows up to about two feet in height and can spread like a weed. Well known for its aromatic menthol aroma, peppermint is widely used in candies and gums. But peppermint has a long history of medicinal use. Peppermint relieves pain, calms spasms, alleviates flatulence, improves digestion, cools the skin, and serves as a general tonic. Native Americans were aware of these, and other, uses. The Shoshone and Paiute have used a tea made from the dried leaves and stems to treat gas pains. The Menominee treat pneumonia by drinking a tea made by combining peppermint with catnip. Most Eastern Woodland tribes boiled mint and inhaled the steam to help relieve head colds, congested lungs, and bronchial and sinus problems. When applied topically, peppermint can help relieve itching and pain.

To make a tea, pour one cup of boiling water over two to three teaspoons of peppermint leaves. Steep for fifteen to twenty minutes and strain. Drink up to two cups a day.

See also BRONCHITIS; CATARRH; COLITIS; COUGHS AND COLDS; DIARRHEA; DYSMENORRHEA; FATIGUE; FLATULENCE; HANGOVER; HEADACHE; HEARTBURN; INDIGESTION; LIVER PROBLEMS; NAUSEA AND VOMITING; NERVOUSNESS; PNEUMONIA; *and* STRESS *in Part Two.*

Pine

Several varieties of pine (*Pinus* sp.) grow in North America and have been used by Native Americans for their lumber, bark, needles, cones, and seeds. However, the white pine (*Pinus strobus*), also called soft pine, seems to be especially beneficial. The white pine is an evergreen tree that can grow more than 150 feet in height. The inner bark of the tree makes an effective expectorant and has a long history of use in treating coughs and colds. The Chippewa have treated cuts and wounds by making a decoction of the trunk bark and combining it with the inner bark of the wild cherry and wild plum. Other tribes have used compresses to treat burns and other injuries.

To make a tea, pour one cup of boiling water over one teaspoon of the inner bark of the white pine. Let steep for several minutes; strain. Take a tablespoon at a time, as needed. You can also make a tea from the needles; take a quarter to half a cup at a time, up to three times a day.

See also COUGHS AND COLDS; DIARRHEA; *and* WOUNDS *in Part Two.*

Pipsissewa

Pipsissewa (*Chimaphila umbellata*) is a perennial evergreen plant that grows around the world in temperate climates. Also called Prince's pine, pipsissewa is an effective diuretic, helpful in treating kidney and bladder problems, a fact many Native American tribes, including the Okanagan-Colville, the Iroquois, and the Delaware, recognized. Pipsissewa has also been used by Native Americans to treat childbirth complications, respiratory problems, rheumatism, stomach cancer, constipation, venereal disease, and heart ailments.

To make a tea, pour one cup of boiling water over two teaspoons of pipsissewa leaves. Let steep for twenty to thirty minutes; strain and cool. Take up to one cup a day, a tablespoon at a time.

See also INTESTINAL WORMS *and* KIDNEY AND BLADDER PROBLEMS *in Part Two.*

Pleurisy Root

Pleurisy root (*Asclepias tuberosa*) is a perennial herb native to North America that grows up to three feet in height. Also called butterfly weed, the root of this plant is an effective expectorant, used to treat colds, bronchial problems, and, of course, pleurisy. The Natchez used a tea made by boiling the roots to treat pneumonia. The Omaha believed this herb so important that only members of the Shell society were allowed to dig and distribute the roots.

Topically, the pulverized root can be applied to cuts, bruises, and other injuries. In fact, the Menominee consider it one of their most important medicines.

To make a tea, place one teaspoon of pleurisy root in a pan and cover with one cup of water. Bring to a boil and boil for twenty to thirty minutes; strain. Take up to two cups a day, a tablespoon at a time.

See also ASTHMA; COUGHS AND COLDS; HEADACHE; NERVOUSNESS; PLEURISY; PNEUMONIA; STRESS; *and* WOUNDS *in Part Two.*

Pulsatilla

Pulsatilla (*Anemone pulsatilla; also Pulsatilla occidentalis*), also called pasque flower and meadow anemone, grows to about eight inches in height and produces violet purple flowers. Pulsatilla is used to treat nervous conditions and fatigue. The Okanogan and Thompson Indians have found it helpful in disorders affecting the digestive and respiratory tracts. An infusion is also beneficial as an eyewash and a topical treatment for rheumatism.

To make a tea, pour one cup of boiling water over one teaspoon of the fresh pulsatilla herb; steep for thirty minutes; strain. Take a tablespoon at a time, up to half a cup per day.

Caution: Avoid this herb if you are pregnant.

See also DYSMENORRHEA; EAR INFECTIONS; FATIGUE; MACULAR DEGENERATION; NERVOUSNESS; *and* PREMENSTRUAL SYNDROME *in Part Two.*

Queen of the Meadow

Queen of the meadow (*Filipendula ulmaria*) is a perennial herb that grows to about six feet in height. Also known as meadowsweet, this herb promotes perspiration so it is helpful in diseases marked by fever. Queen of the meadow can also fight inflammation. The Meskwaki have used it to treat a variety of heart problems. Because it contains salicylic acid (the active ingredient in aspirin), queen of the meadow can be used in much the same way as aspirin.

To make a tea, pour one cup of boiling water over two tablespoons of queen of the meadow. Let steep for ten to fifteen minutes. You can also make a tea from the roots by boiling three tablespoons of the dried root in one cup of water. Take up to one cup a day.

Caution: Avoid this herb if you are allergic to salicylates, such as aspirin.

See also BRONCHITIS; CHICKENPOX; COUGHS AND COLDS; GOUT; *and* KIDNEY AND BLADDER PROBLEMS *in Part Two.*

Raspberry

In addition to its delicious fruit, the raspberry plant (*Rubus idaeus*) has long been used by Native Americans for its healing leaves and roots. This perennial plant grows up to one foot in height and can become quite invasive, much like the blackberry. The Chippewa and Omaha have used raspberry roots to treat bowel trouble such as dysentery and diarrhea. The leaves, however, are also effective, probably because they contain astringent tannins.

Raspberry leaves also contain very high amounts of iron, manganese, and niacin and high quantities of magnesium, selenium, vitamin A, and vitamin C.

To make a tea, pour two cups of boiling water over two tablespoons of raspberry leaves. Let steep for ten to fifteen minutes and strain. Take up to two cups a day.

See also ALZHEIMER'S DISEASE; BRUISES; CANKER SORES; CATARACTS;

Catarrh; Circulatory Disorders; Diarrhea; Dysmenorrhea; Fatigue; Macular Degeneration; Sprains and Strains; *and* Toothache *in Part Two.*

Red Willow

Red willow (*Salix lasiandra*) is a tall (up to fifty feet) tree that grows along streams primarily in the western United States. Native Americans have utilized almost every part of the willow to make everything from baskets to bows to tools to toys. Also called Pacific willow, the inner bark of the tree is used in tonics. In fact, the Okanagan-Colville Indians drank a tea made from the inner bark of the red willow (along with wild cherry bark) as a general illness remedy. The Bella Coola have used it to treat diarrhea, while the Kashaya Pomo treated colds and sore throats with a leaf decoction.

To make a tea, place one teaspoon of the bark in a pan and cover with two cups of water; bring to a boil and boil until reduced to one cup; strain; cool. Take as needed, a half cup at a time up to two cups a day.

See also Malaise *in Part Two.*

Redroot

Redroot (*Ceanothus americanus*) is a deciduous shrub whose root has a red interior, hence its name. Also called New Jersey tea and wild snowball, the root bark of this plant has astringent and sedative properties. Native Americans have used redroot to treat headaches, joint and muscle pain, fevers, and respiratory problems such as coughs, laryngitis, and pneumonia. According to one report, the Seminole used redroot as a hallucinogen to influence speech and awareness.

To make a tea, pour one cup of boiling water over one teaspoon of redroot root bark; steep for thirty minutes; strain. Take a tablespoon at a time, up to two cups a day.

NATIVE
AMERICAN
HERBS

See also BRONCHITIS; LIVER PROBLEMS; MALAISE; *and* PNEUMONIA *in Part Two.*

Rose

Dozens of rose varieties (*Rosa* sp.) grow in North America, and Native Americans learned how to use whatever grew in their region. The leaves, the petals, the hips, and the roots of the rose have been widely used as remedies for a variety of conditions, including colds, fevers, diarrhea, influenza, and stomach trouble.

Tea made from rose hips or roots was used by the Omaha as an eyewash to treat eye inflammations, while a tea from the roots' inner bark was used by the Chippewa in the same manner to treat cataracts. The Flathead and Cheyenne Indians treated snow blindness with an eyewash made by boiling the petals, stem bark, or root bark.

To make a tea, place a handful of rose petals in a glass container and cover with two cups of boiling water; let steep for thirty minutes; strain and cool. Take a quarter cup at a time, as often as desired.

See also CATARACTS *and* SINUSITIS *in Part Two.*

Sage

Sage (*Salvia officinalis*) is a perennial evergreen shrub whose leaves have culinary as well as medicinal value. Although the names are similar, sage is not related to big sagebrush (see Big Sagebrush in this section). Sage can help reduce perspiration (some sources say by as much as 50 percent), so it is helpful in treating conditions such as tuberculosis that are marked by night sweats. Sage also eliminates mucous, so it can improve respiratory conditions. In fact, the Cherokee have used this herb to relieve asthma, coughs, and colds. It also has long been used as a digestive aid (the Cherokee use a leaf infusion to relieve diarrhea). The Mohegan have used sage to treat worms.

To make a tea, pour one cup of boiling water over two teaspoons of dried sage leaves. Let steep for thirty minutes and strain. Take up to two cups a day, a tablespoon at a time. This infusion is also effective as a gargle.

See also Catarrh; Croup; Tonsillitis; *and* Tuberculosis *in Part Two.*

St. John's Wort

St. John's wort (*Hypericum perforatum*) is a perennial shrub that grows up to two feet in height. Used for hundreds of years by the Klamath, Nez Perce, Umatilla, Yakima, and other Native Americans, this herb has a calming effect on the nerves but is also considered by some herbalists to be a stimulant. Currently it is widely used to treat depression. St. John's wort is helpful in alleviating fatigue and also seems effective at relieving menstrual cramping and premenstrual syndrome. There is some evidence that St. John's wort can fight HIV, the virus that causes AIDS.

To make a tea, pour one cup of boiling water over two teaspoons of dried St. John's wort leaves or flowers; steep for ten to fifteen minutes and strain. Drink half a cup in the morning and half a cup at night.

Caution: St. John's wort can cause photosensitivity, so stay out of the sun if you are taking this herb. In addition, caution should be exercised if you are taking a monoamine oxidase (MAO) inhibitor or other antidepressant.

See also Chronic Fatigue Sydrome; Dysmenorrhea; Fatigue; Sunburn; *and* Wounds *in Part Two.*

Sarsaparilla

Sarsaparilla (*Smilax officinalis*) is a perennial vine that grows primarily in the South. The roots and rhizomes from this herb are said to be good for arthritis, coughs and colds, and catarrh. Sarsaparilla has diuretic properties and can also promote perspiration and improve overall health. The Penobscot Indians drank a root tea to treat colds and coughs. Topically, sarsaparilla tea has been used to treat ringworm and other skin problems.

To make a tea, pour one cup of boiling water over one teaspoon of sarsaparilla root. Let steep for thirty minutes and strain. Take up to two cups a day.

See also ARTHRITIS *and* RINGWORM *in Part Two.*

Saw Palmetto

Saw palmetto (*Serenoa serrulata*) is a low-growing shrub. The brownish-black saw palmetto berries have gained a lot of attention in the United States lately as a cure for prostate problems, especially enlargement of the prostate (benign prostatic hyperplasia). The berries are also used to treat respiratory tract problems, including coughs and colds, bronchitis, and asthma. The Seminole Indians have also used the saw palmetto for food, and several tribes have utilized various parts of the plant to make baskets, brooms, and ropes.

Saw palmetto berries contain very high amounts of zinc, a mineral often used to treat prostate problems. The berries are also high in phosphorus, chromium, iron, magnesium, manganese, niacin, potassium, riboflavin, selenium, silicon, and thiamin.

To make a tea, pour two cups of boiling water over two teaspoons of saw palmetto berries; steep for thirty minutes. Drink up to two cups per day.

See also PROSTATE PROBLEMS *in Part Two.*

Self-Heal

Self-heal (*Prunella vulgaris*), also called woundwort and all-heal, is a perennial herb found throughout the United States and used by many tribes. Self-heal has astringent properties, so it is very effective when used internally as a treatment for diarrhea. The Mohegan, Iroquois, and Delaware have used it to relieve fevers. Several tribes, including the Blackfoot, Cherokee, Coast Salish, Iroquois, Quebec Algonquin, Quileute, and Qunault, have used it topically to treat acne, boils, bruises, cuts, hemorrhoids, sores, and other skin inflammations.

To make a tea, pour one cup of boiling water on one teaspoon of self-heal leaves; steep for thirty minutes and strain. Take as needed.

See also DIARRHEA *and* HEARTBURN *in Part Two.*

Seneca Snakeroot

Seneca snakeroot (*Polygala senega*) is a perennial herb native to North America that grows fifteen to eighteen inches in height. The crooked root of this plant resembles a snake, hence its name. Also called senega snakeroot and mountain flax, this herb was introduced to European settlers by the Seneca Indians. Seneca snakeroot is an effective expectorant and is widely used to treat respiratory conditions, such as coughs and colds. Chewing on the root can help relieve a sore throat. Several tribes, including the Seneca, Winnebago, and Dakota have also used the herb topically to treat snakebite.

To make a tea, pour one cup of boiling water over one teaspoon of seneca snakeroot leaves. Let steep for thirty minutes and strain. Take up to one cup a day, a tablespoon at a time.

See also BRONCHITIS; CROUP; SORE THROAT; *and* TONSILLITIS *in Part Two.*

Skullcap

Skullcap (*Scutelleria lateriflora*) is a perennial herb that grows to about three feet in height. It was once called mad dog weed since it was believed to be effective against rabies. Also known as blue pimpernel, skullcap is a sedative, good for treating nervousness, excitability, and insomnia. It also has diuretic properties. Native Americans have also used the plant to promote menstruation.

To make a tea, pour one cup of boiling water over one teaspoon of dried skullcap; steep for twenty to thirty minutes; strain. Take a tablespoon four times daily.

See also NERVOUSNESS *and* STRESS *in Part Two.*

Slippery Elm

Slippery elm (*Ulmus fulva*) is a deciduous tree that grows to fifty feet or more. Also known as the American elm and Indian elm, the inner bark of this tree has soothing properties whether used internally or externally. Several tribes, including the Pillager Ojibwa, Mohegan, and Chippewa, have used slippery elm to treat sore throats. A tea made from the bark also makes an effective laxative.

A paste made from the inner bark has been used topically on boils, wounds, and burns. The Cree used the bark for toothaches, and the Catawba used a salve for rheumatism.

To make a tea, pour one cup of boiling water over two teaspoons of powdered slippery elm inner bark. Let steep for an hour or more and strain. Take two teaspoons an hour, up to two cups a day.

See also AGING; BRONCHITIS; CIRCULATORY DISORDERS; ECZEMA; PSORIASIS; SINUSITIS; SKIN RASH; SORE THROAT; TONSILLITIS; *and* WOUNDS *in Part Two.*

Solomon's Seal

Solomon's seal (*Polygonatum multiflorum*) is a perennial herb that grows up to about three feet in height. Also known as dropberry, this herb is an emetic (induces vomiting), but a decoction of the roots is also used as a tonic. The roots contain allantoin, which has healing and anti-inflammatory properties. Solomon's seal has been used topically on skin blemishes, bruises, and inflammations.

To make a tea, place one teaspoon of Solomon's seal root in a pan; cover with one cup of water; bring to a boil; reduce heat and simmer thirty minutes; cool; strain. Take up to half a cup per day, a tablespoon at a time.

See also BOILS; HEARTBURN; *and* TUBERCULOSIS *in Part Two.*

Speedwell

Speedwell (*Veronica officinalis*) is a creeping perennial plant that only grows about ten inches in height. Also known as gypsy weed, the flowers from this herb make an effective expectorant, so it has been used by the Cherokee to treat coughs and colds. Speedwell has also been used to reduce fevers, while the flowers have diuretic properties. It can be used topically to treat boils and earaches.

To make a tea, pour one cup of boiling water on two tablespoons of flowering speedwell. Steep for thirty minutes and strain. Take up to two cups a day, a tablespoon at a time. This also makes an effective gargle for coughs and colds.

See also CATARRH; COUGHS AND COLDS; GOUT; LIVER PROBLEMS; *and* WOUNDS *in Part Two.*

Stone Root

Stone root (*Collinsonia canadensis*) is a perennial herb that grows to about four feet in height. Also called horseweed and hardhack, this plant's rhizome and dried root are used to treat kidney and bladder problems, as well as gastrointestinal disorders. It is an effective diuretic so it can eliminate excessive water retention as often occurs during and just before menstruation. Stone root is also used as an ingredient in tonics. This herb is also effective when used topically. The Iroquois used the leaves in a poultice to relieve headaches, while the Cherokee made a deodorant from the flowers.

To make a tea, pour one cup of boiling water over one teaspoon of the root; steep for thirty minutes and strain. Take a tablespoon at a time, up to one cup a day.

Caution: Overdoses of this herb can irritate the lining of the intestinal tract, causing nausea and pain; dizziness may also occur.

See also MALAISE *in Part Two.*

Strawberry Leaf

Best known for its fragrant and delicious fruit, the strawberry (*Fragaria* sp.) is a perennial plant that grows wild in many parts of the country. The Blackfoot have used wild strawberry tea to treat diarrhea, while several tribes, including the Ojibwa and Potawatomi, have used the roots to treat stomach problems. Strawberry tea is also used against kidney problems and rheumatoid arthritis.

When used topically, strawberry leaf compresses are effective against rashes, eczema, and acne.

To make a tea, pour one cup of boiling water over two tablespoons of strawberry leaves; steep for thirty minutes until cool and strain. Take whenever needed.

See also DIARRHEA; FATIGUE; GOUT; *and* SKIN RASH *in Part Two.*

Sumac

Sumac (*Rhus glabra*) is a tall shrub or tree that can grow up to twenty feet in height. The Mohegan gargled a tea made from the berries to treat sore throat. Several tribes, including the Osage, Kansas Indians, and Kickapoos, have used the root to stop blood flow. Sumac has also been used to treat dysentery, urinary disorders, and stomach troubles.

To make a tea, pour one cup of boiling water on one teaspoon of sumac bark, berries, or leaves. Let steep for thirty minutes and strain. Take up to two cups a day, a tablespoon at a time.

See also SORE THROAT *and* TONSILLITIS *in Part Two.*

Sunflower

Sunflower (*Helianthus annuus*) is a large flowering plant that can grow several feet in height and have a flower over one foot wide. Sunflower seeds are a good source of protein and are also used to make cooking oil. Sunflowers have been used by Native Americans to treat a variety of skin inflammations. The Meskwaki healed burns by applying a poultice made from sunflowers, while the Hopi used the plant to treat insect bites. The Ojibwa used a sunflower poultice to draw blisters.

To make an infusion, pour one cup of boiling water over one tablespoon of sunflower petals; steep for thirty minutes and strain.

See also BURNS *in Part Two.*

Uva Ursi

The uva ursi (*Arctostaphylos uva-ursi*) is an evergreen shrub whose leaves are used to treat urinary tract infections. Also called bearberry and kinnikinick, this herb has antibacterial activity and has been used by several tribes to treat kidney and liver problems. The Okanagan-Colville Indians drank a tonic for that purpose made by combining the stems and leaves of uva ursi along with twigs from the Oregon grape.

Uva ursi contains tannins and other astringents, flavonoids such as quercetin, and is very high in iron, manganese, and vitamin A.

To make a tea, place one teaspoon of uva ursi leaves in a pan; cover with one cup of water; bring to a boil and boil for fifteen minutes; cool; strain. Take a quarter cup up to three times a day.

Caution: This herb should be avoided by pregnant or nursing women and may cause liver damage in children younger than twelve. In addition, excessive use can cause stomach discomfort and pain.

See also KIDNEY AND BLADDER PROBLEMS *in Part Two.*

Valerian

Valerian (*Valeriana officinalis*) is a hardy perennial herb also known as all-heal and heliotrope. The root of the valerian has a very unpleasant smell but nevertheless is one of the best herbal relaxants, well known for its calming properties. This herb is very effective at treating nervous conditions and insomnia, a fact many Native American tribes have known for centuries. The Blackfoot have also used valerian to treat stomach problems. Several tribes, including the Thompson Indians of British Columbia and the Menominee, have used valerian root topically to treat cuts and wounds.

To make a tea, pour two cups of cold water over one teaspoon of chopped valerian root. Let soak for eight to ten hours. Drink up to one cup per day, either throughout the day, if treating nervousness, or at bedtime, if treating insomnia.

See also Carpal Tunnel Syndrome; Croup; Insomnia; Nervousness; Sinusitis; Sprains and Strains; Stress; *and* Tonsillitis *in Part Two.*

White Cedar Leaf Tips

The white cedar (*Thuja occidentalis*) is a tall tree that normally reaches fifty feet in height, though some exceptional trees can grow much higher. Native to North America, this tree's even-grained aromatic wood is generally resistant to decay and termites. American Indians utilized every part of this tree for a variety of reasons. They made spears and arrows from the wood, they burned the wood for fuel and incense, and they used the leaves and branches as insecticides. They also used the leaves and branches to treat a wide range of diseases. The tips of the leaves can be made into a tea to treat respiratory conditions such as coughs and colds. The cones relieve colic in babies, the needles functioned as a diuretic. Topically, an infusion of the leaves is effective against skin conditions, including athlete's foot and ringworm. Many tribes, including the Ojibwa and the Potawatomi, burned the smoke in purification ceremonies, while the Chippewa burned the incense in religious ceremonies.

To make a tea, pour one cup of boiling water over two teaspoons of leaf tips; steep for ten minutes, until cool, and strain. Take a quarter cup at a time, up to three times daily.

See also ATHLETE'S FOOT; COUGHS AND COLDS; PROSTATE PROBLEMS; *and* RINGWORM *in Part Two.*

White Oak

The white oak (*Quercus alba*) is a deciduous tree that is native to North America. Oak trees can grow quite tall, up to 150 feet in height, although most are 50 to 100 feet tall. Native Americans have used oak for its lumber, as well as for the healing power of its bark and acorns. Oak bark has astringent properties and has been used to treat bowel trouble, intestinal pain, and diarrhea. The Delaware and other tribes have also used bark decoctions to treat sore throats, coughing, and other respiratory problems. Topically, bark decoctions and infusions make good washes for abscesses, sores, and other skin problems.

To make a tea, place one tablespoon of white oak bark in two cups of water. Bring to a boil; reduce heat and simmer for ten minutes; strain and cool. Take up to two cups a day.

See also ABSCESS; BEDSORES; BRUISES; CANKER SORES; COLD SORES; ECZEMA; PSORIASIS; *and* SKIN RASH *in Part Two.*

White Willow

The white willow (*Salix alba*) is a deciduous tree that can grow up to seventy-five feet in height. The bark of the willow has been used to treat pain and fever for thousands of years. The bark contains a phytochemical called salicin, which is closely related to salicylic acid, or aspirin. In fact, aspirin was originally made from the white willow. The Cree, Chippewa, Huron, Mohawk, and other American Indians have used willow bark in much the same way as aspirin to reduce fever, relieve headaches, treat arthritis and other pain, and fight inflammation.

To make a tea, place one to two teaspoons of willow bark in a pan; cover

NATIVE
AMERICAN
HERBS

with one cup of water. Let soak for four to five hours, then gradually bring to a boil; boil thirty minutes; remove from heat; cover; cool and strain. Take up to one cup a day, a tablespoon at a time.

Caution: Individuals who must avoid aspirin should also avoid white willow.

See also ACNE; ARTHRITIS; BITES AND STINGS, INSECTS; BOILS; CARPAL TUNNEL SYNDROME; EAR INFECTIONS; FATIGUE; HEADACHE; PLEURISY; PREMENSTRUAL SYNDROME; SINUSITIS; SPRAINS AND STRAINS; TONSILLITIS; *and* TOOTHACHE *in Part Two.*

Wild Cherry

Wild cherry (*Prunus serotina; P. virginiana*) is a large tree whose bark and root bark have long been used medicinally. Also called chokecherry, the twigs, roots, and fruit of this plant have been used by American Indians to treat diarrhea, lung congestion, coughs, and colds. There are a number of cough remedies on the market, including cough syrup and lozenges, that contain wild cherry bark. Tea made from the inner bark has also been used to treat sore throats, sores, burns, wounds, and conjunctivitis. The Okanagan-Colville make a general tonic from the wild cherry branches. For many tribes, the cherries were a key ingredient in pemmican, a dried mixture of fruit, meat, and fat.

To make a tea, pour one cup of boiling water over one teaspoon of the wild cherry bark; steep for thirty minutes; cool and strain. Take a tablespoon at a time, every half hour, as needed.

Caution: Excessive intake of wild cherry bark can cause difficulty breathing, spasms, and twitching. Wild cherry bark contains a cyanidelike chemical called hydrocyanic acid.

See also ARTHRITIS, CANCEROUS TUMORS; COUGHS AND COLDS; CROUP; KIDNEY AND BLADDER PROBLEMS; MALAISE; PNEUMONIA; SORE THROAT; TONSILLITIS; *and* WOUNDS *in Part Two.*

Wild Indigo Root

The wild indigo root (*Baptisiae tinctoria*) is a perennial herb that grows to about four feet in height. Also known as horsefly weed and indigo broom, the root of this plant has been used as an antiseptic wash to treat skin sores, eczema, and wounds. Wild indigo also acts as an emetic and a stimulant.

To make a tea, pour two cups of boiling water over one teaspoon of wild indigo root. Let steep for fifteen to twenty minutes and strain. Take one teaspoon at a time, as needed.

Caution: Use caution with this herb, as excessive intake can be poisonous. Authorities do not agree, however, on how much is excessive.

See also BURNS; SINUSITIS; *and* TONSILLITIS *in Part Two.*

Wild Plum

Wild plum (*Prunus americana*) is a tree native to North America. The plum fruit is normally small and hard and often used as a laxative. The Cheyenne, however, have used a tea made from the roots to treat diarrhea. The roots of the plant have also been used by the Chippewa to treat worms. The Meskwaki found that a tea made from the bark was effective at relieving stomach problems and vomiting. The Omaha and Meskwaki have treated wounds by applying decoctions made from the root bark.

To make a tea, place one teaspoon of the root in a glass container and cover with two cups of water; allow to soak overnight; strain. Take a quarter cup at a time, three times a day.

See also WOUNDS *in Part Two.*

Wintergreen

Wintergreen (*Gaultheria procumbens*) is an aromatic evergreen shrub native to North America. Also called Canada tea and deerberry, wintergreen is often used to relieve pain and inflammation. The leaves of the wintergreen contain methyl salicylate, which is closely related to aspirin. Several tribes, including the Delaware and the Mohican, have used a tea made from the leaves to treat kidney disorders. The Great Lakes and Eastern Woodland Indian tribes have used poultices from wintergreen, applying them topically to treat arthritic aches and pains.

To make a tea, pour one cup of boiling water over one teaspoon of wintergreen leaves. Let steep for up to twenty minutes and strain. Drink two tablespoons at a time, up to one cup per day.

See also ASTHMA; CRAMPS, MUSCLE; HEADACHE; HEARTBURN; *and* SPRAINS AND STRAINS *in Part Two.*

Witch Hazel

Witch hazel (*Hamamelis virginiana*) is a deciduous shrub also called tobacco wood. Many tribes, including the Cherokee and Iroquois, have used a tea made from the leaves or bark to treat coughs, colds, fevers, and sore throats. Because witch hazel is an astringent, it is also effective at treating diarrhea. Topically, witch hazel is widely used to treat skin irritations, bites and stings, cuts, and bruises and is an ingredient in many over-the-counter topical medicines.

To make a tea, place one teaspoon of witch hazel bark or leaves in a pan; cover with one cup of water; bring to a boil; boil for ten to fifteen minutes; cover; cool and strain. Take up to one cup a day, a tablespoon at a time.

See also BRUISES; CATARRH; CHICKENPOX; DIARRHEA; HEARTBURN; SINUSITIS; SORE THROAT; TONSILLITIS; VARICOSE VEINS; *and* WOUNDS *in Part Two.*

Yarrow

Yarrow's Latin name, *Achillea millefolium*, is derived from the name of the Greek hero best known for his vulnerable heel. A perennial herb, yarrow is also called milfoil, nosebleed, and soldier's woundwort; the latter two terms giving a good indication of yarrow's wound-healing abilities. Yarrow is also effective at treating catarrh, coughs, colds, and fever. In fact, many tribes, including the Cheyenne, Menominee, Lakota, Assiniboin, Gros Ventre, and Okanagan, have used the herb for one or more of these conditions.

Sometimes the use of an herb seems contradictory; such is the case with yarrow. The Iroquois drank a tea made from yarrow root to treat diarrhea, while the Okanagan combined yarrow root with other herbs to treat constipation. Yarrow can encourage the flow of bile, so it improves digestion.

Many tribes have used yarrow topically in compresses to treat bleeding; as washes for skin irritations such as burns, eczema, hives, and poison ivy; and as poultices to treat wounds.

To make a tea, pour one cup of boiling water over one tablespoon of dried yarrow. Let steep for twenty to twenty-five minutes and strain. Take up to one cup a day, a tablespoon at a time.

See also BITES AND STINGS, INSECT; CATARRH; COUGHS AND COLDS; DIARRHEA; FATIGUE; LIVER PROBLEMS; VARICOSE VEINS; *and* WOUNDS *in Part Two.*

Yellow Dock

Yellow dock (*Rumex crispus*) is a perennial herb that has been used medicinally for thousands of years. Also called curled dock and rumex, this herb is used as a laxative and a tonic. The Iroquois have used a tea from the roots to treat upset stomachs, kidney problems, and general bowel problems. Many tribes, including the Blackfoot, Paiute, and Shoshone, have used the herb topically, applying the mashed root to sores and swellings.

Yellow dock is very high in manganese, phosphorus, and vitamin A and high in calcium, iron, magnesium, riboflavin, selenium, thiamin, and vitamin C.

To make a tea, place one teaspoon of yellow dock root in a pan; cover with one cup of water; bring to a boil and boil for twenty to thirty minutes. Take up to two cups a day, as needed.

Caution: Excessive intake of yellow dock can irritate the intestinal tract.

See also ACNE; DIARRHEA; ECZEMA; HEARTBURN; LIVER PROBLEMS; MEASLES; MONONUCLEOSIS; PSORIASIS; RINGWORM; SKIN RASH; *and* STEAT-ORRHEA *in Part Two.*

Yerba Mansa

Yerba mansa (*Anemopsis californica*) is a creeping perennial herb that grows from one to two feet in height. Native to the southwestern United States, this plant is used as an antiseptic, both internally and topically. Also known as yerba del manzo and swamp root, this herb can help soothe coughs and colds and has been used for such a purpose by the Cahuilla, Kawaiisu, Pima, Taba-tulabal, and others. It can also relieve the pain of skin ulcers when used as a bark infusion, leaf infusion, or poultice.

To make a tea, place a teaspoon of the dried root in a container and cover with one cup of cold water. Let soak overnight and then strain. Take a quarter to half a cup, up to four times daily.

See also ABSCESS; BOILS; CANKER SORES; COLD SORES; COUGHS AND COLDS; CRAMPS, MUSCLE; NAUSEA AND VOMITING; PROSTATE PROBLEMS; SINUSITIS; *and* SPRAINS AND STRAINS *in Part Two.*

Yerba Sante

Yerba sante (*Eriodictyon californica*) is an aromatic evergreen shrub that grows to about six to seven feet in height and is native to the western part of North America. Also called mountain balm and bearsweed, this herb is used to treat coughs, colds, and other respiratory problems, as well as fevers. Many tribes dried and then smoked the leaves of the herb as a treatment for asthma and lung congestion.

To make a tea, pour one cup of boiling water over one teaspoon of yerba sante leaves; steep for thirty minutes and strain. Take up to half a cup a day, a tablespoon at a time.

See also ALLERGIES; ASTHMA; COUGHS AND COLDS; SORE THROAT; *and* TONSILLITIS *in Part Two.*

Yucca

Yucca (*Yucca glauca*) is a tall (up to ten feet in height) evergreen plant whose roots are used to relieve pain in conditions such as arthritis, gout, and rheumatism. Also called small soapweed, the roots and leaves of the plant are commonly used to make a diuretic. Yucca has also been widely used as a food source. Many tribes, including the Navajo, Lakota, and Cheyenne, have also made soap and shampoo from yucca leaves, while the Blackfoot, Kiowa, and others used the roots in a tonic to treat hair loss.

To make a tea, pour one cup of boiling water over one teaspoon of pulverized yucca roots; steep for thirty minutes and strain. Take as needed, half a cup at a time, up to two cups a day.

See also ARTHRITIS *and* HAIR LOSS *in Part Two.*

Herbs Not Recommended for Use

While you may have seen some of the following herbs recommended in other books, I advise against using them, as they are toxic. While they have a long history of use in Native American healing and may be included in Native American herbal formulas and well-respected books on Native American herbs, recent studies have found, unfortunately, that these herbs have toxic effects in the body. They should therefore not be used; if absolutely necessary, they should be used only under the close supervision of a well-trained herbal expert. ☠

♠ Adder's-tongue (*Erythronium americanum*) is a perennial herb native to the eastern United States. Also called dog-tooth violet, serpent's tongue, and yellow snowdrop, adder's-tongue was used internally to treat a variety of conditions ranging from vomiting to hiccups and externally in a poultice for ulcers, tumors, abscesses, skin inflammations, and hives. However, even a small amount of the bulb (one to two grams) will produce vomiting. Weiner states that adder's-tongue may contain the alkaloid colchine, and the fresher the plant, the higher the colchine content. Colchine is extremely toxic, so anyone taking adder's-tongue internally would be advised to use only minute amounts. Adder's-tongue was listed in the *United States Pharmacopoeia* between 1820 and 1863 as a treatment for gout. ☠

♠ Bitterroot (*Apocynum androsaemifolium* and *A. cannabinum*) is also called dogbane, dog's bane, milk weed, and westernwall. Although bitterroot was widely used by many tribes to treat numerous conditions, including sore throats, colds and coughs, constipation, and convulsions, it contains cymarin, a poisonous glycoside. Nevertheless, some Native Americans drank a bitterroot tea once a week as an oral contraceptive. The Chippewa used a decoction of the dried root to treat heart palpitations, while the Potawatomi used it as a cardiac treatment and diuretic. Because it is poisonous, and also because of its heart-stimulating properties, bitterroot is now considered too toxic to ingest. ☠

♠ Bloodroot (*Sanguinaria canadensis*) is also called red puccoon, Indian plant, and tetterworth. The root of this plant has been used extensively by numerous Native American tribes. Many tribes used bloodroot to treat respiratory problems and digestive problems. The Chippewa mixed it with blue cohosh to treat digestive cramps. Topically, it has been used to treat ringworm, nasal polyps, and skin burns, and it appears to have been an effective insect repellent. Unfortunately, we now know that bloodroot is toxic (it contains the poisonous alkaloid sanguinarine, as well as other alkaloids). In fact, it is classified as unsafe by the Food and Drug Administration (FDA). Bloodroot acts as a narcotic and an emetic, but higher doses can irritate the mucous membranes and result in diarrhea, intestinal colic, and vomiting, and can lead to total collapse. ☠

♠ Henbane (*Hyoscyamus niger*), also called devil's eye and stinking nightshade, is a biennial herb. Used by Native Americans to treat insomnia and convulsions, and to induce hypnosis (as a hallucinogen), henbane is now classified as an unsafe herb. ☠

♠ Jimsonweed (*Datura stramonium*) is an annual herb that grows nearly everywhere in North America. Also called mad-apple, this plant has been used by Native Americans for its hypnotic, sedative, and hallucinogenic properties. Unfortunately, jimsonweed is also poisonous. According to noted herb expert James Duke, jimsonweed is so toxic that it has been used in suicides and homicides. ☠

♠ Mandrake (*Podophyllum peltatum*), also called May apple and raccoon berry, has been used by Native Americans to treat bladder and liver problems, asthma, insomnia, and worms. However, mandrake is a dangerous and poisonous plant. ☠

♠ Mescal beans (*Sophora secundiflora*) have been used for their hallucinogenic properties, but the seeds and the flowers are poisonous. ☠

♠ Mistletoe (*Phoradendron serotinum*), or American mistletoe, is an evergreen shrub used to induce labor and cause abortion. All parts, but especially the berries, are poisonous. ☠

♠ Peyote (*Lophophora williamsii*) is a cactus used as a hallucinogen. Peyote's active constitute is mescaline, which stimulates the respiratory system and the heart. Peyote is a narcotic hallucinogen and should be used with extreme care. ☠

♠ Sassafras (*Sassafras officinalis; S. albidum*) is a deciduous tree whose bark has been used by Native Americans as a tonic, as well as to treat kidney problems, bronchitis, and fever. Sassafras is toxic to the liver and, in fact, is considered carcinogenic and should be avoided. ☠

♠ Tansy (*Tanacetum vulgare*) is an aromatic, perennial herb also known as bitter buttons. Tansy tea has been used to treat constipation, fever, and worms; to promote menstruation; and to induce abortion. Tansy is considered toxic and poisonous and should be avoided. Note: The toxic properties of tansy can be absorbed through the skin, so avoid topical application. ☠

♠ Wormwood (*Artemisia absinthium*), also called absinthe, has been used by Native Americans to treat indigestion and other stomach problems, induce abortion, eliminate worms, and fight coughs and colds. However, wormwood depresses the central nervous system and is considered an unsafe herb. Wormwood is an ingredient in the French liqueur absinthe, which was outlawed in France in the early 1900s. ☠

PART TWO

Healing Indian Formulas for Individual Conditions

In Part Two, you will read about disorders and symptoms that can be relieved or at least helped with herbs traditionally used by Native Americans. Consider this book to be your Native American herb bible. But keep in mind that, because herbs were the first medicines, they can sometimes be very powerful. Do not gather herbs from the wild unless you know what you are doing. And please, grow your own herbs whenever possible; native herbs are becoming increasingly rare, and many are threatened with extinction.

Choosing the right herbs and herbal combinations for your health needs is most important for you. Follow three easy steps to identify and satisfy your herbal and nutritional needs:

1. Identify the injury or disorder that is affecting you.

2. Identify the areas of your health status and specific needs that require additional support.

3. Choose the most appropriate treatment program from this book

that fits your needs. This should include herbs, enzymes, vitamins, minerals, and phytochemicals.

As always, if you are pregnant or nursing, if you suffer from a chronic condition such as heart disease or diabetes, or if you are currently taking medications of any kind, please consult with your physician or a well-trained herbal specialist before self-treating. Herbs and other supplements can alter the way your body utilizes other medicines. They can sometimes improve the efficacy of medicines and, at other times, interfere with the absorption or action of a particular drug.

If you have any questions about the appropriateness of any treatment, seek the services of a well-trained health-care professional. This book and the formulas contained herein are not intended to replace the services of a well-trained health-care professional. ⌐

Abrasions

(*See* Wounds)

Abscess

An abscess is a local accumulation of pus. It can occur almost anywhere on or in the body, but it most frequently occurs on the skin and on the gums of the mouth. Abscesses can be very tender and painful and are marked by inflammation, swelling, heat, redness, and often fever. Abscesses are caused by an infection, so orthodox medical doctors often treat them with antibiotics. But herbs are an effective and safe alternative, without the side effects of antibiotics.

SKIN-ABSCESS–FIGHTING TEA

> *30 drops echinacea tincture (See Part One for directions for tinctures.)*
> *60 drops yerba mansa tincture*
> *1 cup warm water*

Combine all the ingredients. Take up to five times per day to stimulate the immune system and help eliminate the infection.

A TOPICAL WASH FOR SKIN AND GUM ABSCESSES

1 to 2 teaspoons barberries
1 tablespoon white oak bark
1 teaspoon echinacea root
1 teaspoon granulated Oregon grape root
2 cups boiling water

Combine the herbs in a glass container. Pour the boiling water over the herbs and soak for 3 to 4 hours; strain. Use three times a day as a wash. If you are using this tea to treat a gum abscess, be sure to swish the liquid around in your mouth for several minutes before spitting it out.

See also BARBERRY; ECHINACEA; OREGON GRAPE; WHITE OAK; *and* YERBA MANSA *in Part One.*

Acne

Acne is an inflammatory skin condition that commonly affects adolescents (because of increased glandular activity during the teen years). Acne occurs when the sebaceous glands, which are located just beneath the skin, become inflamed. These glands secrete an oil called sebum, which acts to lubricate the skin. Acne results when the pores of the skin become clogged by the sebum. Acne can occur any time in life and may be due to allergies, high-sugar or high-fat diets, heredity, the use of oral contraceptives and other drugs (such as cortisone), hormone changes, and stress.

In addition to the herbs listed in the recipes below, other herbs that are helpful in fighting the inflammation that occurs with acne include bur-

HEALING
INDIAN
FORMULAS
FOR INDIVIDUAL
CONDITIONS

89

dock, dandelion, echinacea, and ginger root (all used topically and internally), and *Ginkgo biloba,* ginseng, licorice, and white willow bark (all used internally).

ACNE-FIGHTING TEA

⅓ cup Oregon grape root tea (page 60)
50 drops yellow dock tincture

Combine the ingredients. Take up to one-third of the mixture three times daily.

ACNE WASH

1 cup horsetail tea (page 51)
30 drops gotu kola tincture

Combine ingredients in a glass container with a lid. Use as much as needed to wash the skin, three times daily.

See also BURDOCK; DANDELION; ECHINACEA; GINGER; GINKGO BILOBA; GINSENG; GOTU KOLA; HORSETAIL; LICORICE; OREGON GRAPE; WHITE WILLOW; *and* YELLOW DOCK *in Part One.*

Aging

We all want to live to a ripe old age without looking a day over twenty-nine! Unfortunately, aging is a fact of life that occurs as the body's ability to function declines. The process of aging—marked by wrinkles, aching joints, fatigue, and loss or graying of hair—is accelerated by a poor diet, lack of exercise, excessive exposure to sunlight's ultraviolet rays, and lifestyle choices including smoking and drug use. These and other factors increase free-radical activity. Free radicals are highly unstable molecules that damage the cells' DNA and interfere with the cells' ability to function. A number of herbs function as antioxidants, which effectively eliminate free radicals. These herbs include Ginkgo biloba, ginger, parsley, and milk thistle. Other herbs contain flavonoids, naturally occurring compounds that can improve the strength of your body's capillaries (tiny blood vessels), and therefore your circulation (something that is often impaired as we age). These herbs include berries, cherries, black currants, elderberries, horsetail, and milk thistle.

AGING TEA #1

½ cup Ginkgo biloba *tea (page 45)*
½ cup ginseng tea (page 50)

Combine the ingredients. Take one-third of a cup three times daily. Ginkgo is known to improve memory, while ginseng can boost energy levels.

AGING TEA #2

5 drops cayenne tincture
30 drops burdock tincture
15 drops goldenseal tincture
10 drops ginger root tincture
½ cup slippery elm tea (page 72)
1 cup warm water

Combine all ingredients. Take 2 to 3 tablespoons three times per day to improve circulation.

See also BLACK CURRANT; BURDOCK; CAYENNE; ELDER; GINGER; *GINKGO BILOBA*; GINSENG; GOLDENSEAL; HORSETAIL; MILK THISTLE; PARSLEY; *and* SLIPPERY ELM *in Part One; and* ARTHRITIS, CATARACTS, CIRCULATORY DISOR-

DERS, CONSTIPATION, MACULAR DEGENERATION, PROSTATE PROBLEMS, *and* VARICOSE VEINS *in Part Two.*

Allergies

An allergy is a hypersensitive reaction to any of a number of substances. Allergies occur when the body's immune system malfunctions, going into "overdrive" to help protect the body from a substance it sees as foreign. Allergies are very common in the United States. In fact, more than one-third of all Americans suffer from an allergy of one type or another. Common symptoms include nasal congestion, coughing, watery eyes, sneezing, fatigue, and headaches. Some allergies may cause hives or an itchy rash. Severe allergies can cause the blood pressure to drop to dangerously low levels, leading to anaphylactic shock and death.

Hay fever is an acute type of allergy usually caused by airborne pollens. Trees and grasses are the typical culprits in this condition. Symptoms of hay fever include itchy eyes, mouth, and throat; watery eyes; sneezing; nasal discharge; and headaches.

Some people are allergic to molds, pollens, and dusts. Others react to certain foods such as wheat, milk, peanuts, eggs, or shellfish. Certain cosmetics or chemicals and even bee stings bring grief to many. The best way to treat an allergy is to avoid the offending substance. When that isn't possible, herbs can help check the watery eyes, nasal discharge, and coughing that occur with some allergies.

In addition to those herbs listed in the recipes below, other helpful herbs for allergies include agrimony, goldenseal, ground ivy, and marigold.

 ALLERGY TEA #1

1 teaspoon barberry root

1 teaspoon Oregon grape root

1 cup water

Combine the herbs in a pan and cover with the water. Bring to a boil. Reduce heat and simmer for 30 minutes. Strain. Take one-third cup three times daily.

ALLERGY TEA #2

1 teaspoon oxeye daisy leaves
1 teaspoon pearly everlasting flowers
1 teaspoon yerba sante leaves
3 cups boiling water

Combine the herbs in a glass container and cover with the water; steep for 30 minutes; strain. To use, take one-half to one cup every six hours.

ALLERGY TEA #3

2 tablespoons nettle leaves
1 teaspoon Oregon grape root
2 cups boiling water

Combine all the herbs in a glass container and cover with the water; steep for 30 minutes; strain. Take one-quarter cup three times a day.

See also AGRIMONY; BARBERRY; GOLDENSEAL; GROUND IVY; MARIGOLD; NETTLE; OREGON GRAPE; OXEYE DAISY; PEARLY EVERLASTING; *and* YERBA SANTE *in Part One.*

Alzheimer's Disease

Alzheimer's disease (AD) is a type of dementia in which parts of the brain atrophy and cease to function. Named after Dr. Alois Alzheimer, the German physician who first discovered the condition, AD is marked by tangled fibers and plaques in the brain. Alzheimer's patients suffer from memory loss and a decline in language skills and may have difficulty completing even the simplest tasks. There may be many factors involved in Alzheimer's disease development, but researchers know there is a genetic factor in many cases. Head injury, exposure to certain toxins, and even viruses and nutritional deficiencies may also be implicated in some cases of AD.

Helpful herbs for Alzheimer's disease include *Ginkgo biloba* and gotu kola, which can enhance blood circulation; and raspberries and black currants, which contain anthocyanidins, known to fight free radicals, reduce blood vessel plaque formation, and maintain capillary blood flow.

ALZHEIMER'S TEA #1

> *2 teaspoons* Ginkgo biloba *leaves*
> *2 tablespoons gotu kola*
> *2 cups boiling water*

Combine the herbs in a glass container and cover with the water; steep for 30 minutes; strain. Take one-quarter cup three times a day.

ALZHEIMER'S TEA #2

> *2 tablespoons raspberry leaves*
> *2 teaspoons black currant leaves*
> *2 cups boiling water*

Combine the herbs in a glass container and cover with the water. Steep for 30 minutes. Strain. Take half a cup several times a day.

See also BLACK CURRANT; *GINKGO BILOBA*; GOTU KOLA; *and* RASPBERRY *in Part One.*

Anemia

Anemia is a blood disorder marked by either red blood cells containing too little hemoglobin or too few red blood cells in the blood. (Hemoglobin is the protein in red blood cells that carries oxygen.) Anemia can have a number of causes, including alcoholism, excessive bleeding, illness, infections, poor bone marrow function, poor diet, and pregnancy. It is important to determine the cause of the anemia and treat the underlying condition.

ANEMIA TEA

2 teaspoons barberry root

2 teaspoons Oregon grape root

4 tablespoons nettle leaves

2 cups cold water

Combine the herbs in a glass container. Cover with the water. Soak overnight. Strain. Take up to one-half cup three times daily.

See also BARBERRY; NETTLE; *and* OREGON GRAPE *in Part One.*

Arthritis

There are two types of arthritis: rheumatoid arthritis and osteoarthritis. Rheumatoid arthritis (RA) is an autoimmune condition where the body sees itself as the enemy. The immune system's antibodies attack the joints and soft tissues, causing inflammation, pain, and gradual deterioration of the joint. RA can be a debilitating condition, especially when it occurs in young children.

Osteoarthritis is a degenerative disease, also called wear-and-tear arthritis. This form of arthritis affects many of us as we age. It occurs as the joints wear out over time. It usually starts in the joints of the hands and feet but eventually can affect even the larger joints of the body. Both rheumatoid arthritis and osteoarthritis can cause pain and stiffness.

In addition to the herbs listed below, other beneficial herbs for arthritis include bilberry, black currant, nettle, and vervain. The following treatments are effective for both osteoarthritis and rheumatoid arthritis.

ARTHRITIS TEA #1

2 teaspoons devil's claw tuber
3 teaspoons white willow bark
1 teaspoon feverfew herb
2 teaspoons yucca root
2 teaspoons sarsaparilla root
3 cups cold water

Combine the herbs in a glass container and cover with the water. Soak overnight. Drain. Take one-half cup three times daily.

ARTHRITIS TEA #2

25 drops black cohosh tincture
90 drops wild cherry bark tincture
90 drops mullein tincture
1 cup warm water

Combine the above herbs in a glass container and cover with the water. Take one-third of the mixture three times daily.

ARTHRITIS TEA #3

1 teaspoon black cohosh root
1 teaspoon chamomile flowers
1 teaspoon cascara sagrada bark
2 cups water

Combine the above herbs in a glass container; cover with the water; stir thoroughly to combine. Place 1½ teaspoons of the mixture in one cup boiling water; steep for 10 minutes; strain. Take one cup in the morning and one in the evening.

ARTHRITIS OINTMENT

1 pound petroleum jelly
1 tablespoon Canada balsam
2 tablespoons cayenne
2 tablespoons chamomile

Melt one pound of petroleum jelly in a double boiler. Add herbs; stir; heat for 2 hours. Remove from heat and strain by pouring the mixture through a cheesecloth, squeezing the cloth to release all the liquid. While warm, pour the ointment into glass containers; cool. Apply topically, as needed for arthritis pain.

See also BALSAM BILBERRY; BLACK COHOSH; BLACK CURRANT; BLUE VERVAIN; CASCARA SAGRADA; CAYENNE; CHAMOMILE; DEVIL'S CLAW; FEVERFEW; MULLEIN; NETTLE; SARSPARILLA; WHITE WILLOW BARK; WILD CHERRY; *and* YUCCA *in Part One.*

Asthma

If you've ever heard a child with asthma fighting for breath, you'll never forget the wheezing sound or the panic you feel as his or her skin begins to turn blue from lack of oxygen. Asthma is actually a common lung disease that affects people of all ages. In this disease, the trachea and bronchial tubes become inflamed. This causes the airways to narrow, restricting the flow of air, which in turn leads to shortness of breath, difficulty breathing, coughing, wheezing, and a tightness in the chest. An asthma attack can last from a few minutes to a few days and, if severe, can be life threatening.

No cause for the asthma can be determined for many people; however, for others, asthma attacks can be brought on by allergies to molds, pollen, or other allergens, as well as certain foods and drugs. Asthma can also be triggered by cold, damp weather; inhaling dust, smoke, or other irritants; and even infections. Unfortunately, asthma is on the upswing in this country, possibly because of the irritants in our polluted air.

In addition to the herbs in the following recipes, other helpful herbs include coltsfoot, echinacea, ginseng, goldenseal, passionflower, pleurisy root, wintergreen, and yerba sante.

ASTHMA TEA #1

1 teaspoon elecampane root
2 teaspoons horehound herb
1 teaspoon blue vervain leaves
2 cups water

Combine the herbs in a pan and cover with water. Bring to a boil; reduce heat and simmer for about 20 minutes; strain and cool. Drink up to two cups a day, a mouthful at a time.

ASTHMA TEA #2

2 teaspoons powdered Indian root
2 teaspoons granulated echinacea root
2 teaspoons elecampane root
2 cups water

Combine the herbs in a pan and cover with the water. Soak for several hours; strain. Take one-half cup two times daily.

See also Blue Vervain; Coltsfoot; Echinacea; Elecampane; Ginseng; Goldenseal; Horehound; Indian Root; Passionflower; Pleurisy Root; Wintergreen; *and* Yerba Sante *in Part One.*

Athlete's Foot

Athlete's foot (*tinea pedis*) is a fungal skin infection that is very common. It usually occurs between the toes and sometimes on the soles of the feet. It is marked by a rash and skin redness. Athlete's foot can be very painful and itchy and, in some cases, may result in blisters. It is caused by a fungus that thrives in moist, warm places, such as showers. It is also very contagious and can be acquired through contact with infected shoes, shower floors, or pool surfaces.

Athlete's foot usually improves with good hygiene. Wash the affected area well with soap and water and dry completely (using a hair dryer is a good idea). In addition to the following formula, a wash made with marigold and pau d'arco is also helpful for this condition.

ATHLETE'S FOOT TOPICAL WASH

4 teaspoons big sagebrush root
4 teaspoons white cedar leaf tips
2 cups water

Combine the herbs in a nonmetallic container and cover with the water. Soak for 8 hours; strain. Apply the liquid topically several times a day.

See also Big Sagebrush; Marigold; Pau d'arco; *and* White Cedar Leaf Tips *in Part One.*

Back Pain

Back pain affects most of us at some time in our lives. It can be a dull ache or a sharp burning and stabbing. Sometimes back pain is accompanied by pain that radiates down your leg. This is called sciatica and is a sign that pressure is being placed on the nerves of the spinal cord. Sometimes back pain can be so severe that it limits your activities and renders you bedridden. Often, relaxing the muscles of the back can relieve back pain.

In addition to those herbs listed in the recipes below, other beneficial herbs include barberry, black cohosh, black currant, black haw, blue cohosh, devil's claw, echinacea, feverfew, and blue vervain.

BACK PAIN TEA #1

2 teaspoons crampbark
2 teaspoons kava kava root
2 cups water

Combine the herbs in a pan and cover with water. Bring to a boil; reduce heat; simmer for 30 minutes. Cool and strain. Take up to one cup per day. This tea can help relieve sciatic pain.

BACK PAIN TEA #2

1 teaspoon coltsfoot leaves
2 teaspoons St. John's wort leaves
2 cups boiling water

Combine the herbs in a glass container and cover with boiling water; steep for 15 to 30 minutes; strain. Take one-half cup in the morning and one-half cup at night.

SECRETS
OF NATIVE
AMERICAN
HERBAL
REMEDIES

100

BACK PAIN TEA #3

1 teaspoon chopped valerian root
2 teaspoons white willow bark
2 cups cold water

Combine the herbs in a pan and cover with the water. Soak overnight; strain. Take up to one cup a day, a tablespoon at a time. This tea can help relieve pain caused by nerve irritation.

See also BARBERRY; BLACK COHOSH; BLACK CURRANT; BLACK HAW; BLUE COHOSH; BLUE VERVAIN; COLTSFOOT; CRAMPBARK; DEVIL'S CLAW; ECHINACEA; FEVERFEW; KAVA KAVA; ST. JOHN'S WORT; VALERIAN; *and* WHITE WILLOW *in Part One.*

Bedsores

A bedsore, also called a *decubitus ulcer*, is an area of damage to the skin that can occur when pressure is applied to an area of the body for a prolonged period of time. The pressure restricts blood flow to the area and also causes irritation, leading to sores.

Skin ulcers are raw, open sores that occur when the top layer of skin cracks and peels away. They are marked by swelling, redness, pain, heat, and inflammation. They may also be infected and full of pus. Bedsores are very common in individuals in casts, as well as those confined to wheelchairs or to bed. In fact, the most common sites for bedsores are the lower back, the buttocks, and the heels. Some authorities estimate that treating bedsores and other decubitus ulcers costs the nation over $1 billion every year.

Other herbs beneficial for treating skin conditions such as bedsores include burdock, evening primrose, and nettle.

BEDSORE TOPICAL WASH

2 teaspoons marigold flowers

1 teaspoon granulated echinacea root

1 tablespoon white oak bark

2 cups water

Combine the herbs in a glass container and cover with the water; soak overnight; strain. Use as a wash periodically throughout the day.

See also BURDOCK; ECHINACEA; EVENING PRIMROSE; MARIGOLD; NETTLE; *and* WHITE OAK *in Part One.*

Bites and Stings, Insect

Some time during our lives, most of us will be bitten or stung by a mosquito, bee, wasp, ant, spider, tick, or more exotic creature, such as a snake or jelly-fish. We call it a "bite," but most insects and other creatures puncture the skin rather than actually take a bite. It is the substance the animal leaves in the wound and not the wound itself that usually does the damage.

Bites and stings frequently cause localized itching, pain, swelling, and red-ness. If untreated, any bite or sting can fester and become infected. Even though itching may be severe, resist the urge to scratch, as a secondary infec-tion could result.

Native Americans have had thousands of years to practice using herbs on snakebites. Some of the most helpful herbs for this condition include echi-nacea and Seneca snakeroot.

In addition to those herbs listed below, other helpful herbs for treating insect bites and stings include black currant, ginger, *Ginkgo biloba*, licorice, and white willow.

Note: If you are stung by a bee or other pest and begin to feel weak, or if you notice any swelling anywhere on the body, call a physician immediately. You

SECRETS
OF NATIVE
AMERICAN
HERBAL
REMEDIES

102

may be allergic to the sting and need emergency medical attention. Needless to say, if you are stung by a rattlesnake or other venomous snake, get immediate medical care.

TOPICAL WASH FOR BITES AND STINGS

2 teaspoons comfrey leaves
2 tablespoons marshmallow leaves
1 tablespoon dried yarrow
1 cup boiling water

Combine the herbs in a nonmetallic container and cover with boiling water. Steep for 15 to 30 minutes; strain. Use as a topical wash.

STING-HEALING OINTMENT

1 pound petroleum jelly
4 teaspoons dried agrimony leaves
4 teaspoons dried marigold flowers

Melt petroleum jelly in a double boiler. Stir in the herbs and heat for 2 hours until the herbs begin to get crispy. Strain by pouring through cheesecloth. Squeeze the cloth to release all the liquid. While warm, pour the ointment into clean glass containers. Use as needed.

See also AGRIMONY; BLACK CURRANT; COMFREY; GINGER; *GINKGO BILOBA*; LICORICE; MARIGOLD; MARSHMALLOW; WHITE WILLOW; *and* YARROW *in Part One.*

Boils

A boil is a raised and swollen sore caused by a staphylococcal bacterial infection that enters the skin through the hair follicles. Boils usually have a yellow or white center and are rimmed in red. It may look like a very bad pimple and

HEALING
INDIAN
FORMULAS
FOR INDIVIDUAL
CONDITIONS

103

can be very painful. Several boils appearing together in a cluster are called a carbuncle. Boils appear most frequently on the face, neck, armpits, and in the groin.

In addition to those herbs listed below, other helpful herbs include *Ginkgo biloba*, ginger root, licorice, marigold, marshmallow, Solomon's seal, and white willow bark.

A HEALING TEA

30 drops echinacea tincture
60 drops yerba mansa tincture
1 cup warm water

Combine the above ingredients in the warm water in a nonmetallic container. Take up to five times per day to stimulate the immune system and help eliminate the infection.

A TOPICAL WASH

½ cup barberry tea (page 21)
½ cup white oak tea (page 77)
½ cup echinacea tea (page 41)
½ cup Oregon grape root tea (page 60)

Combine the above ingredients in a glass container with a lid. Use three times a day as a topical skin wash.

See also BARBERRY; ECHINACEA; GINGER; *GINKGO BILOBA*; LICORICE; MARIGOLD; MARSHMALLOW; OREGON GRAPE; SOLOMON'S SEAL; WHITE WILLOW; *and* YERBA MANSA *in Part One.*

SECRETS
OF NATIVE
AMERICAN
HERBAL
REMEDIES

104

Bronchitis

Bronchitis is an inflammation of the bronchial tubes that can range from a mild case (much like a bad cold) to a severe case, leading to pneumonia. Bronchitis may be accompanied by a fever, severe coughing, thick sputum, difficulty breathing, chills, and a sore throat. Bronchitis usually is caused by an infection but can also occur after inhaling dust, smoke, or other irritants. Repeated bouts of bronchitis can lead to chronic bronchitis, in which the bronchial tubes may become permanently damaged.

In addition to those herbs listed below, other helpful herbs include echinacea, black elder, Canadian fleabane, horehound, licorice, peppermint, queen of the meadow, seneca snakeroot, and slippery elm.

BRONCHITIS TEA #1

2 teaspoons black cohosh root

2 teaspoons powdered Indian root

2 teaspoons chamomile flower

2 cups water

Honey, to taste

Combine the above herbs in a pan; cover with the water. Bring to a boil; reduce heat and simmer for 30 minutes; strain. Add honey if desired. Take one tablespoon in two cups of water several times a day.

BRONCHITIS TEA #2

1 teaspoon marshmallow leaves or flowers

1 teaspoon coltsfoot leaves

1 teaspoon mullein leaves and flowers

½ cup boiling water

Honey

HEALING
INDIAN
FORMULAS
FOR INDIVIDUAL
CONDITIONS

105

Combine the above herbs; steep one teaspoon of the mixture in the boiling water; strain. Sweeten with honey. Take one-half cup, three or four times a day, hot.

BRONCHITIS TEA #3

1 teaspoon elecampane root
2 tablespoons nettle leaves
1 cup boiling water

Combine the above herbs. Pour the boiling water over the herbs and steep for 30 minutes; strain. Sweeten with honey, if desired. Take up to two cups a day.

BRONCHITIS TEA #4

1 to 2 slices of fresh ginger root
1 teaspoon pearly everlasting flowers or leaves
1 teaspoon redroot
1 cup boiling water

Combine the above herbs; steep in the boiling water for 30 thirty minutes; strain. Take one-half cup of the tea, three times daily.

See also Black Cohosh; Black Elder; Canadian Fleabane; Chamomile; Coltsfoot; Echinacea; Elecampane; Ginger; Horehound; Indian Root; Licorice; Marshmallow; Mullein; Nettle; Pearly Everlasting; Peppermint; Queen of the Meadow; Redroot, Seneca Snakeroot; *and* Slippery Elm *in Part One.*

Bruises

A bruise occurs when the tissue that lies just beneath the skin is injured. Caused by trauma of some kind, the injury ruptures the capillaries (small

SECRETS
OF NATIVE
AMERICAN
HERBAL
REMEDIES

106

blood vessels) causing bleeding under the skin. This, in turn, leads to the characteristic black-and-blue appearance of bruises. In addition to the characteristic discoloration, bruises can cause pain and swelling in the affected area. Some people bruise for no obvious reason. This is usually a sign of capillary fragility, that is, the capillary walls are weak and easily rupture. This can occur for a number of reasons, including aging, diabetes, alcoholism, and nutritional deficiencies.

CAPILLARY TEA

2 teaspoons dried black currant leaves
2 tablespoons raspberry leaves
1 tablespoon white oak bark
2 cups water

Combine the above herbs in a pan and cover with the water. Bring to a boil; reduce heat and simmer for 20 minutes; cool; strain. Take up to two cups a day. This tea will help strengthen the capillaries.

TOPICAL BRUISE TREATMENT

1 teaspoon witch hazel bark
1 cup water
2 teaspoons dried hyssop

Place the witch hazel in a pan and cover with the water; bring to a boil; boil for several minutes; cover; cool and strain. To the resulting liquid, add the dried hyssop and soak for 8 hours; strain. Use this solution topically, as needed.

See also BLACK CURRENT; HYSSOP; RASPBERRY; WHITE OAK; *and* WITCH HAZEL *in Part One.*

HEALING
INDIAN
FORMULAS
FOR INDIVIDUAL
CONDITIONS

107

Burns

A burn is an injury to the skin or other tissues caused by fire (or another form of heat), electricity, chemicals, or radiation. Burns are classified according to their severity as first-degree, second-degree, or third-degree. In a first-degree burn, the skin will turn red and swell but will not blister. In a few days, there is complete healing, without scarring. The damage from a second-degree burn goes much deeper. The skin turns very red and there is blistering, although the skin heals without scarring. The most severe burn, third-degree, penetrates the skin, destroying both the epidermis and dermis (the segment of the skin beneath the epidermis). A third-degree burn can result in scar tissue formation. Burn tissue can become necrotic and also develop into a serious infection. Skin elasticity can be destroyed. A third-degree burn may actually be less painful than a more superficial first- or second-degree burn because nerve endings in the skin are destroyed. Burns can also occur internally from swallowing very hot liquids or inhaling hot air (such as that from a fire).

A severe burn can cause dangerous systemic damage, such as respiratory tract injury, infection, and shock. Anyone suffering from a severe burn should seek immediate medical attention to counter these potentially life-threatening effects. Herbs, however, can help relieve the pain from a minor burn and encourage rapid healing.

BURN POULTICE

1 tablespoon dried coneflower flowers
1 tablespoon dried hyssop flowers
1 tablespoon dried goldenrod flowers
1 tablespoon dried sunflower petals

Combine the above ingredients; moisten with boiling water and place between two layers of cheesecloth; let cool, and apply to the affected area. When dry, remoisten. Use as often as necessary.

SECRETS
OF NATIVE
AMERICAN
HERBAL
REMEDIES

108

IMMUNITY STRENGTHENER

30 drops echinacea tincture

20 drops wild indigo root tincture

1 cup warm water

Combine the above herbs in the warm water; take up to five times a day. A burn can weaken the body, leaving you vulnerable to illness and infection. Use this tea to strengthen immunity.

See also CONEFLOWER; ECHINACEA; GOLDENROD; HYSSOP; SUNFLOWER; and WILD INDIGO ROOT *in Part One.*

Cancerous Tumors

Tumors can occur anywhere in the body, including the brain, breast, colon, lung, pancreas, prostate, and rectum, or on the skin itself. Cancer is the common name for a malignant tumor. The term *cancer* refers not just to one disease, but rather a constellation of more than 100 different diseases.

Cancer is marked by an uncontrolled growth and spread of abnormal cells. Normally, the body forms new cells only when needed to replace damaged or old cells (it does this through a highly controlled process called "cell division," when one existing cell divides into two cells). Children and infants produce new cells for repair and to complete their growth and development. However, if cells multiply uncontrolled, a tumor develops. As the tumor grows, it can interfere with organ function, leading to death. Tumors are either benign (harmless) or malignant (cancerous).

Anyone suffering from cancer of any kind should be under a physician's care. Herbs can help improve appetite and serve as supportive cancer therapy. But be sure to let your doctor know if you are using herbs, as they can increase the efficacy of some drugs, while reducing the efficacy of others.

HEALING
INDIAN
FORMULAS
FOR INDIVIDUAL
CONDITIONS

APPETITE ENHANCER

1 teaspoon angelica root

1 teaspoon ginseng root

2 cups boiling water

Combine the above herbs and cover with the boiling water; steep for 30 minutes; strain. Take two teaspoons, four times a day. Other herbs that improve appetite include devil's claw, ginger, horehound, and mirabilis.

SUPPORTIVE CARE

1 teaspoon Canadian fleabane leaves

2 tablespoons Oregon grape root

1 teaspoon echinacea root

2 tablespoons wild cherry bark

2 cups water

Place the above herbs in a pan; cover with the water. Bring to a boil and boil for 20 to 30 minutes; cool and strain. Take twice a day, a tablespoon or two at a time.

See also ANGELICA; CANADIAN FLEABANE; DEVIL'S CLAW; ECHINACEA; GINGER; GINSENG; HOREHOUND; MIRABILIS; OREGON GRAPE; *and* WILD CHERRY *in Part One.*

Candidiasis

Candidiasis is a yeast infection caused by *Candida albicans*. Candida, found in the vagina, in the digestive tract, and on the skin, is normally harmless. However, for a variety of reasons, including antibiotic use, hormonal changes,

SECRETS
OF NATIVE
AMERICAN
HERBAL
REMEDIES

110

poor diets, and diminished immunity, candida can grow out of control and cause infections of the mucous membranes and the skin. Vaginal infections, also called yeast infections, are often caused by candida and can be very uncomfortable. This condition is marked by vaginal itching, an abnormal vaginal discharge, pain, redness, and inflammation. It may also be painful to urinate.

In addition to the following formula, a marigold and echinacea infusion used as a douche can also be beneficial for candidiasis.

CANDIDIASIS TEA

1 tablespoon pau d'arco bark
2 teaspoons big sagebrush root
1 cup water

Combine the above ingredients in a glass container and cover with the water; soak overnight; strain. Take one-half cup up to three times a day.

See also BIG SAGEBRUSH; ECHINACEA; MARIGOLD; *and* PAU D'ARCO *in Part One.*

Canker Sores

Canker sores are small sores usually found on the lining of the mouth, although they can also occur on the lips, on the tongue, or in the throat. Also called aphthous ulcers, they can be white or yellow and are surrounded by red, inflamed tissue. These small ulcers can be extremely painful for several days and may be accompanied by fever and swollen lymph glands. Canker sores can be brought on by stress, viral infections, poor dental hygiene, and nutrient deficiencies. Injuries (such as certain dental procedures) can also cause canker sores to develop.

In addition to those herbs listed below, other helpful herbs include raspberries and black currants, which contain anthocyanidins, helpful in fighting inflammation.

A TOPICAL WASH

½ cup barberry tea (page 21)
½ cup white oak tea (page 77)
½ cup echinacea tea (page 41)
½ cup Oregon grape root tea (page 60)

Combine the above ingredients in a glass container with a lid. Use three times a day as a mouthwash. Be sure to swish the liquid around in your mouth for several minutes.

SKIN ABSCESS TEA

30 drops echinacea tincture
60 drops yerba mansa tincture
1 cup warm water

Combine the above herbs in the warm water in a nonmetallic container. Take up to five times per day to stimulate the immune system.

See also BARBERRY; BLACK CURRANT; ECHINACEA; OREGON GRAPE; RASPBERRY; WHITE OAK; *and* YERBA MANSA *in Part One.*

Carbuncles

(*See* Boils)

SECRETS
OF NATIVE
AMERICAN
HERBAL
REMEDIES

112

Cardiovascular Disorders

(*See* Circulatory Disorders)

Carpal Tunnel Syndrome

Carpal tunnel syndrome (CTS) is a condition marked by sometimes severe pain in the wrists and hands. There may also be numbness, a burning sensation, wrist inflammation, swelling, and wrist weakness in either or both hands. The bones of the wrist (called the *carpus*) form a tunnel through which nerves pass. Pain and swelling occur when these nerves and the nerves that pass between the tendons of the forearm muscles are compressed. Carpal tunnel syndrome usually occurs in individuals who do repetitive hand and wrist movements, such as typists, tennis players, grocery store clerks, and the like. It is most common in women between the ages of thirty and sixty, but it can affect anyone at any time.

Several diseases and conditions are also associated with carpal tunnel syndrome, such as diabetes, thyroid disorders, kidney failure, obesity, rheumatoid arthritis, and high blood pressure.

PAIN TEA

1 teaspoon chopped valerian root
2 teaspoons white willow bark
2 cups cold water

Combine the herbs in a pan and cover with the cold water. Soak overnight; strain. Take up to one cup a day, a tablespoon at a time. This tea can help relieve nerve pain.

See also VALERIAN *and* WHITE WILLOW *in Part One; and* ARTHRITIS; CIRCULATORY DISORDERS; DIABETES; KIDNEY AND BLADDER PROBLEMS; *and* OBESITY *in Part Two.*

HEALING
INDIAN
FORMULAS
FOR INDIVIDUAL
CONDITIONS

113

Cataracts

A cataract is a "clouding" of the lens of the eye that causes progressively blurred vision. The severity varies depending on the location in the eye and the thickness of the cataract. The thicker a cataract, the more vision will be affected. Cataracts are usually painless, which is why routine visual examinations are so important. Cataracts are the leading cause of blindness in the world. Unfortunately, we don't yet know what causes cataracts, although they can result from several diseases (including diabetes) and from exposure to X rays and sunlight. Cataracts usually occur with aging, but, very rarely, they are present at birth or develop in young people.

CATARACT WASH

½ cup rose petals
2 tablespoons raspberry leaves
2 cups boiling water

Combine the herbs and cover with two cups of boiling water in a nonmetallic container; steep for 15 minutes; cool; strain. Use as an eyewash.

See also RASPBERRY *and* ROSE *in Part One.*

Catarrh

Catarrh is an old-fashioned term, not used much today, that means inflammation of the mucous membranes of the head and throat, accompanied by a discharge (postnasal drip) of runny or viscous fluid, usually from the nose. A person with hay fever or other allergies, bronchitis, asthma, or certain viral infections might suffer from catarrh. In addition to the herbs listed below, other helpful herbs include bilberry, blackberry, black currant, Canadian fleabane, cayenne, coltsfoot, comfrey, echinacea, feverfew, goldenrod, marigold,

SECRETS
OF NATIVE
AMERICAN
HERBAL
REMEDIES

114

marshmallow, oxeye daisy, raspberry, sage, speedwell, vervain, and witch hazel.

CATARRH TEA #1

1 teaspoon boneset
3 teaspoons peppermint leaves
2 tablespoons elder flowers
1 tablespoon yarrow
2 cups boiling water

Combine the herbs and cover with the boiling water in a nonmetallic container; steep 30 minutes, cool, and strain. Take up to two cups a day.

CATARRH TEA #2

2 teaspoons agrimony leaves
1 teaspoon bee balm leaves
1 cup boiling water

Combine the herbs and cover with the boiling water; steep 30 minutes, cool, and strain. Take up to two cups per day.

See also AGRIMONY; BEE BALM; BILBERRY; BLACK CURRANT; BLACK ELDER, BLACKBERRY; BLUE VERVAIN; BONESET; CANADIAN FLEABANE; CAYENNE; COLTSFOOT; COMFREY; ECHINACEA; FEVERFEW; GOLDENROD; MARIGOLD; MARSHMALLOW; OXEYE DAISY; PEPPERMINT; RASPBERRY; SAGE; SPEEDWELL, WITCH HAZEL; *and* YARROW *in Part One; and* ALLERGIES; ASTHMA; *and* BRONCHITIS *in Part Two.*

Chickenpox

Chickenpox is a viral infection marked by a skin rash. The rash (of small red marks) can be very itchy and can appear anywhere on the body. There may

HEALING
INDIAN
FORMULAS
FOR INDIVIDUAL
CONDITIONS

115

also be headache, fever, and loss of appetite (the symptoms tend to be worse in newborns and adults than in children). Chickenpox is highly contagious but is not considered serious for most people, although it can lead to pneumonia. It has historically been a very common childhood disease, but vaccinations have reduced its incidence. A related disease, shingles (herpes zoster), occurs when the virus reactivates itself in the body, usually many years after the initial chickenpox infection. Shingles can be extremely painful. Check with a herbalist about any treatment for children.

CHICKENPOX TEA

2 tablespoons queen of the meadow
1 teaspoon coltsfoot leaves
2 teaspoons marigold flowers
2 cups boiling water

Combine the above herbs and cover with the boiling water in a nonmetallic container; steep for 15 minutes, cool, and strain. Take up to one cup a day, a tablespoon at a time.

TOPICAL WASH

2 tablespoons marigold flowers
1 teaspoon witch hazel leaves
1 cup cold water

Combine the herbs and soak in the cold water overnight; strain. This solution can help relieve the itching of chickenpox.

See also COLTSFOOT; MARIGOLD; QUEEN OF THE MEADOW; *and* WITCH HAZEL *in Part One.*

SECRETS
OF NATIVE
AMERICAN
HERBAL
REMEDIES

116

Chronic Fatigue Syndrome

Chronic fatigue syndrome (CFS) is a confusing condition marked by persistent, debilitating, and profound exhaustion. There also may be fever, sore throat, painful lymph nodes, headaches, sleeping problems, and muscle aches. Other symptoms include confusion, depression, forgetfulness, and irritability. CFS is difficult to diagnose because these symptoms can be signs of numerous other conditions, as well. Because diagnosis is so difficult, the Chronic Fatigue and Immune Dysfunction Syndrome Association of America, Inc. has established criteria to determine whether a person is suffering from CFS:

1. Clinically evaluated, unexplained, relapsing, or persistent chronic fatigue that is not lifelong, but rather of new or definite onset. The fatigue must not be substantially alleviated by rest, not be the result of ongoing exertion, and must result in a substantial reduction of the person's activities (educational, personal, occupational, and/or social).

2. The individual must have at least four of the following symptoms: substantial impairment in concentration or short-term memory; tender lymph nodes; sore throat; multijoint pain with redness or swelling; muscle pain; headache of a new type, severity, or pattern; malaise after exercise that lasts more than twenty-four hours; and unrefreshing sleep. These symptoms must all have occurred after the extreme fatigue was noted and must have recurred or persisted during six or more consecutive months of illness. Of course, other possible causes of the fatigue must also have been ruled out.

CFS is a complex condition whose exact cause is not known, although it seems to involve a dysfunction of the immune system. In some individuals, it begins after an infection with the Epstein-Barr virus, herpes, mononucleosis, or cytomegalovirus.

FATIGUE TEA

1 teaspoon ginkgo biloba *leaves*
½ teaspoon *mirabilis root*
1 teaspoon *ginseng leaves*

HEALING
INDIAN
FORMULAS
FOR INDIVIDUAL
CONDITIONS

117

½ teaspoon pulsatilla leaves

1 tablespoon gotu kola

1 teaspoon St. John's wort

3 cups boiling water

Combine the above herbs in a nonmetallic container, and pour the boiling water over them. Steep for 20 minutes, cool, and strain. Take up to half a cup a day.

See also GINKGO BILOBA; GINSENG; GOTU KOLA; MIRABILIS; PULSATILLA; and ST. JOHN'S WORT in Part One.

Circulatory Disorders

The list of circulatory disorders is almost endless and includes heart disease, strokes, hypertension, and atherosclerosis, to name a few. These and other circulatory conditions are the number-one cause of death in this country, killing nearly one million Americans every year.

As we age, our body's ability to keep a proper equilibrium between blood clotting and blood liquefaction begins to go awry. On the one hand, blood must clot if we are to keep from bleeding to death, yet, on the other hand, it must be free flowing and liquid in order to travel easily through the body's blood vessels. The older we get, the "stickier" our blood gets, and our blood's ability to flow diminishes. When this occurs, the stage is set for blood clots, clogged arteries, strokes, and heart attacks.

In addition to those herbs listed below, other beneficial herbs include black currants and raspberries (which contain anthocyanidins known to reduce blood vessel plaque formation and maintain blood flow in capillaries) and gotu kola.

SECRETS
OF NATIVE
AMERICAN
HERBAL
REMEDIES

118

CIRCULATORY TEA #1

1 teaspoon burdock root

1 teaspoon goldenseal root

1 teaspoon cayenne

2 teaspoons slippery elm bark

2 slices ginger root

3 cups boiling water

Combine the above herbs in a nonmetallic container, and pour the boiling water over them. Steep for 30 minutes, cool, and strain. Take up to one cup a day, two tablespoons at a time.

CIRCULATORY TEA #2

2 teaspoons black cohosh root

4 teaspoons ginkgo biloba *leaves*

2 cups boiling water

Combine the above herbs in a nonmetallic container, and pour the boiling water over them. Soak for 30 minutes, cool, and strain. Take two to three tablespoons at a time, up to six times a day.

FOR ARTERIOSCLEROSIS

2 to 3 ginger slices

2 teaspoons Ginkgo biloba *leaves*

1 teaspoon ginseng leaves

2 cups boiling water

Combine the herbs in a nonmetallic container and cover with the boiling water. Steep for 30 minutes, cool, and strain. Take up to half a cup per day.

See also BLACK COHOSH; BLACK CURRANT; BURDOCK; CAYENNE; GINGER; *GINKGO BILOBA*, GINSENG; GOLDENSEAL; GOTU KOLA; RASPBERRY; *and* SLIPPERY ELM *in Part One.*

Cirrhosis

(*See* Liver Problems)

Cold Sores

Cold sores are small, painful, fluid-filled blisters on the mouth caused by the herpes simplex virus. Tingling, itching, and burning may give you a warning that a cold sore is about to erupt. The blisters may appear a few hours or days after the initial warning signs. After a few days, they eventually dry and form a crust. They usually completely heal within a week or two.

COLD SORE TEA

1 teaspoon burdock root
1 teaspoon dried and powdered goldenseal root
1 cup boiling water
Honey, to taste

Combine the above herbs in a glass container. Pour the boiling water over the herbs; steep for 30 minutes, cool, and strain. You may want to sweeten with honey. Take up to one cup a day.

COLD SORE WASH

1 teaspoon echinacea root
1 teaspoon yerba mansa root
1 tablespoon white oak bark
1 cup boiling water

SECRETS
OF NATIVE
AMERICAN
HERBAL
REMEDIES

120

Combine the herbs in a glass container. Pour the boiling water over the herbs. Steep 30 minutes, cool, and strain. Use the solution as a wash to treat cold sores.

See also BURDOCK; ECHINACEA; GOLDENSEAL; WHITE OAK; *and* YERBA MANSA *in Part One.*

Colds

(*See* Coughs and Colds)

Colitis

Colitis is a type of inflammatory bowel disease (IBD) that refers to inflammation of the colon (Crohn's disease is another type of IBD). Colitis is marked by inflammation and ulceration of the colon (the large intestine). Symptoms include abdominal cramping, fever, and bloody diarrhea with mucus. The diarrhea that accompanies colitis can lead to dehydration. Colitis may occur suddenly or come on gradually. Most cases of colitis begin before an individual is thirty years of age, although it can occur at any time. Colitis has no known cause but is believed to be an autoimmune disorder.

COLITIS TEA #1

1 teaspoon Canadian fleabane leaves
1 cup boiling water
20 drops ocotillo bark tincture

Place the fleabane leaves in a glass jar; pour the boiling water over them; steep for 30 minutes, cool, and strain. Add the ocotillo bark tincture. Take up to one cup per day, a tablespoon at a time.

HEALING
INDIAN
FORMULAS
FOR INDIVIDUAL
CONDITIONS

121

COLITIS TEA #2

1 teaspoon bayberry bark
4 teaspoons peppermint leaves
1 cup water

Combine the herbs in a nonmetallic container, and cover with the water. Bring to a boil; reduce heat; simmer for 30 minutes; cool; strain. Take one to two cups per day.

See also BAYBERRY; CANADIAN FLEABANE; OCOTILLO BARK; *and* PEPPERMINT *in Part One.*

Conjunctivitis

Conjunctivitis (also known as pinkeye) is a very common disorder caused by inflammation of the conjunctiva, the membrane that covers the eyeball and lines the underside of the eyelids. Conjunctivitis is marked by eye pain and burning, eye redness, blurry vision, sensitivity to light, and a gritty, dry feeling in the eyes. There also may be a sticky discharge from the eye. Usually caused by a virus (such as the ones that cause the common cold or measles) or a bacteria, it can also occur because of exposure to irritants or allergens. Conjunctivitis is very easily spread to other people, so avoid touching the affected eye and wash your hands frequently. Children with conjunctivitis should be under the care of a qualified health-care practitioner.

CONJUNCTIVITIS EYEWASH

2 teaspoons chamomile flowers
1 teaspoon Oregon grape root
2 cups boiling water

SECRETS
OF NATIVE
AMERICAN
HERBAL
REMEDIES

122

Combine the herbs. Pour the boiling water over the herbal mixture and steep for 10 to 15 minutes, cool, and strain. Use as an eyewash.

See also CHAMOMILE *and* OREGON GRAPE *in Part One.*

Constipation

Formerly called "costiveness," constipation refers to any irregularity in, or absence of, bowel movements. The frequency of bowel movements depends on your diet, your physical makeup, and your physical habits. Most people have one movement a day, but some people may go two days or more and not suffer from constipation. However, the longer waste products remain in the colon, the more water will be absorbed, and the drier and more compact the waste will become.

Constipation can occur because of a poor diet, inadequate water intake, nervous tension, insufficient exercise, drug use, poor or inconsistent toilet habits, and laxative overuse. A number of diseases, including thyroid problems, circulatory disorders, and colon disturbances (such as fistulas, inflammation, polyps, obstructions, and tumors) can also cause constipation.

In addition to the herbs found in the following formulas, other helpful herbs to relieve constipation include barberry, chicory, marshmallow, and sunflower.

CONSTIPATION TEA #1

One large handful of boneset flowers
One large handful of dandelion flowers
4 ounces cascara bark
2 quarts water
Honey

Combine the above herbs in a pan and cover with two quarts of water; bring to a boil; boil until the mixture reduces to one quart; strain.

Take one cup before breakfast and one at bedtime. You may want to add honey to sweeten.

CONSTIPATION TEA #2

2 teaspoons cascara sagrada
3 to 4 slices ginger root
1 teaspoon cayenne
1 teaspoon Oregon grape root
2 cups boiling water

Combine the above herbs in a pan and cover with two cups of boiling water; steep for 30 to 45 minutes, cool, and strain. Take one table-spoon at a time, up to two cups per day.

See also BONESET; CASCARA SAGRADA; CAYENNE; DANDELION; GINGER; *and* OREGON GRAPE *in Part One.*

Coughs and Colds

The common cold is an upper respiratory tract infection caused by one of more than 100 viruses. Symptoms of a common cold include watery eyes, runny or stuffy nose (rhinitis), head congestion (with a mild, moderate, or severe headache), fatigue, sneezing, and coughing. The cough that often accompanies a cold is the body's attempt to clear the air passage of mucus, dust, or other substances that cause irritation. Your sense of taste and smell may be decreased, and you may run a fever or suffer from chills. A general aching feeling of discomfort and listlessness (malaise) may be present. There may be a sore throat, ranging from mild to severe, as the cold develops. Any or all of these symptoms may be present.

In addition to those herbs listed in the following formulas, several other helpful herbs, including black currant, chamomile, *Ginkgo biloba,* Indian root, peppermint, and queen of the meadow, can help strengthen the immune

SECRETS
OF NATIVE
AMERICAN
HERBAL
REMEDIES

124

system and fight off colds and other viral infections and relieve their symptoms.

COUGH SYRUP #1

2 teaspoons coltsfoot leaves
1 tablespoon wild plum root
2 teaspoons mullein leaves
2 cups boiling water
1 pound honey

Combine the above herbs in the boiling water; in a nonmetallic container steep for 30 minutes and strain. Add one pound of honey, heating and stirring until the honey is dissolved; cool and store in a glass container. Take one tablespoon at a time, as needed.

COUGH AND COLD FORMULA #1

30 drops echinacea tincture
20 drops wild indigo root tincture
2 cups white cedar leaf tips tea (page 76)

Combine the above ingredients and take half a cup at a time, hot, up to three times a day.

LAKOTA COUGH AND COLD FORMULA

1 teaspoon goldenseal root
1 teaspoon mullein leaves
1 teaspoon osha root
1 teaspoon pleurisy root
1 teaspoon yerba mansa root
2 teaspoons yerba sante leaves
2 cups boiling water

Combine the above herbs and cover with the boiling water; steep for 30 minutes, cool, and strain. Take two tablespoons at a time, as needed, up to two cups a day.

LUMBEE COUGH AND COLD FORMULA

3 teaspoons goldenrod leaves
4 teaspoons horehound leaves
2 teaspoons white pine inner bark
4 cups boiling water

Combine the above herbs in a cheesecloth; tie closed with a string. Place the bag in the boiling water; boil for 15 minutes; cool; remove the bundle. Take half a cup of the hot mixture at a time, as needed, up to two cups a day.

COUGH AND COLD FORMULA #2

4 teaspoons agrimony leaves
2 teaspoons mullein leaves
2 teaspoons blue vervain leaves
1 teaspoon oxeye daisy
3 teaspoons horehound leaves
2 teaspoons speedwell
2 cups boiling water

Combine the above herbs in a nonmetallic container and cover with the boiling water; steep for 30 minutes, cool, and strain. Take a table-spoonful every three hours, as needed, up to two cups a day.

COUGH AND COLD FORMULA #3

2 teaspoons boneset herb
2 teaspoons licorice root
2 to 3 slices ginger root

SECRETS
OF NATIVE
AMERICAN
HERBAL
REMEDIES

126

2 teaspoons wild cherry bark
2 cups boiling water

Combine the above herbs in a nonmetallic container and cover with the boiling water; steep for 30 minutes, cool, and strain. Take one to two tablespoons at a time, up to two cups a day, as needed, for a dry tickling cough.

COUGH AND COLD FORMULA #4

2 slices fresh ginger
2 teaspoons pleurisy root
1 cup boiling water

Combine the herbs in a glass container; pour one cup of boiling water over the herbs; steep for 30 minutes, cool, and strain. Take a tablespoon at a time, up to two cups a day. This tea is good for bronchial congestion.

COUGH AND COLD FORMULA #5

1 teaspoon elderflowers
1 teaspoon yarrow flowers
1 cup boiling water

Combine the herbs in a nonmetallic container and cover with one cup of boiling water; steep for 20 minutes and strain. Drink hot every two hours, as needed.

MULLEIN COUGH SYRUP

1 cup of mullein tea (page 58)
1 pound honey

Combine the above ingredients in a pan and heat until the honey is liquid. Remove from heat, cool, and pour into a glass container. Take a tablespoon at a time, as needed.

ELECAMPANE COUGH SYRUP

2 cups of elecampane tea (page 42)
1 pound honey

Combine the tea with the honey and heat on low. Stir to dissolve the honey; when dissolved, remove the mixture from the heat. When cool, pour into glass containers and seal. Take two tablespoons at a time, as needed, up to one cup a day.

HOREHOUND LOZENGES

1½ cups horehound leaves
1½ cups water
3 cups sugar
3 tablespoons corn syrup

Place the horehound leaves in a pan and cover with the water. Bring the mixture to a boil and boil for 20 minutes. Remove from the heat and cool. Strain the solution and add the sugar and corn syrup. Place back on the heat, bring to a boil, then reduce heat to medium. Cook until the mixture reaches 300°F (hard-crack stage). Pour the syrup onto a large buttered baking sheet; cool, then break into one-inch pieces. Use as you would any cough drop.

See also AGRIMONY; BLACK CURRANT; BLACK ELDER; BLUE VERVAIN; BONESET; CHAMOMILE; COLTSFOOT; ECHINACEA; ELECAMPANE; GINGER; *GINKGO BILOBA*; GOLDENROD, GOLDENSEAL; HOREHOUND; INDIAN ROOT; LICORICE; MULLEIN; OSHA ROOT; OXEYE DAISY; PEPPERMINT; PINE; PLEURISY ROOT; QUEEN OF THE MEADOW; SPEEDWELL; WHITE CEDAR LEAF TIPS; WILD CHERRY; WILD INDIGO; YARROW; YERBA MANSA; *and* YERBA SANTE *in Part One; and* BRONCHITIS; CROUP; PLEURISY; PNEUMONIA; SORE THROAT; *and* TONSILLITIS *in Part Two.*

SECRETS
OF NATIVE
AMERICAN
HERBAL
REMEDIES

128

Cramps, Muscle

Cramping muscles are involuntary muscle contractions. They can be very painful and tight. Muscle cramps can be caused by cold temperatures, dehydration, overexercise, nutrient imbalances, and restricted blood flow to the muscles. Muscle cramps also can be caused by an imbalance in the body's electrolytes (electrolytes in the body include calcium, magnesium, potassium, and sodium). Muscle cramps usually occur in the legs, where they can often be severe enough to keep you from walking. Muscle cramps can also occur in the arms, the back, and in virtually any and every muscle of the body.

TOPICAL OINTMENT

20 drops yerba mansa tincture
4 ounces wintergreen oil
1 pound petroleum jelly

Thoroughly mix the above herbs with the petroleum jelly. Use as an ointment to relieve muscle cramps.

MUSCLE CRAMP TEA

2 teaspoons black cohosh root
1 tablespoon ginseng root
2 cups water

Combine the above herbs in a pan and cover with two cups of water; bring to a boil; reduce heat and simmer for 30 minutes, cool, and strain. Take two to three tablespoons up to six times a day.

See also BLACK COHOSH; GINSENG; WINTERGREEN; *and* YERBA MANSA *in Part One; and* DYSMENORRHEA *in Part Two.*

Croup

Croup is an acute inflammation of the respiratory tract and is usually caused by a virus, although allergies and trauma can also bring on an attack, as can anything (such as small objects) that interferes with the airway. The inflammation that occurs with croup causes swelling, which makes breathing difficult. This is why those with the malady make such a loud, barking, labored sound when inhaling. Croup usually occurs in small children (up to age three), although it can occur later. It seems to be worse at night and usually begins with a barking cough and hoarseness. This can progress to respiratory distress that, in some cases, can be quite severe. Fever may accompany the breathing difficulties. Children with croup should be under the care of a qualified health-care practitioner.

CROUP TEA

2 teaspoons elecampane root
2 teaspoons Seneca snakeroot
2 teaspoons sage
2 cups water

Combine the above herbs in a pan and cover with the water; bring to a boil; reduce heat, and simmer for 30 minutes; cool and strain. Take as needed.

CROUP TEA

1 teaspoon mullein leaves
2 teaspoons chopped valerian root
1 teaspoon passionflower
2 teaspoons wild cherry bark
2 cups boiling water

Combine the herbs in a glass container and cover with the boiling water; steep for 30 minutes; cool and strain. Take as needed.

SECRETS
OF NATIVE
AMERICAN
HERBAL
REMEDIES

130

See also ELECAMPANE; MULLEIN; PASSIONFLOWER; SAGE; SENERA SNAKE-ROOT; VALERIAN; *and* WILD CHERRY *in Part One; and* COUGHS AND COLDS *in Part Two.*

Cuts

(*See* Wounds)

Dermatitis

(*See* Eczema)

Diabetes

Diabetes is a condition marked by high levels of sugar (glucose) in the blood. Our bodies use the hormone insulin to promote the entry of glucose into cells. Diabetes occurs when glucose can't enter the cells either because we don't produce enough insulin or don't properly use what we produce.

There are two types of diabetes, Type I and Type II. In Type I, the pancreas produces no insulin at all. This type of diabetes usually develops before an individual reaches thirty and is believed to occur when the body's antibodies attack and destroy the cells of the pancreas that are responsible for producing insulin. Individuals with Type I diabetes require insulin injections. The other type of diabetes, Type II, occurs when the body's insulin production is impaired or when the effectiveness of the insulin produced is decreased. Type II usually occurs in people over the age of thirty, which is why it is often called "adult-onset" diabetes. Proper diet and medications are often sufficient to manage Type II diabetes. The symptoms of both types of diabetes are similar and include frequent urination, extreme hunger, excessive thirst, unusual weight loss, extreme fatigue, and irritability. Cuts and bruises may take a long time to heal, and there may be blurred vision and tingling or numbness in the hands or feet. Women may also suffer from recurrent vaginal infections.

HEALING
INDIAN
FORMULAS
FOR INDIVIDUAL
CONDITIONS

131

It is important to adequately monitor and treat diabetes, because the complications of diabetes are many and can be very serious. Diabetes impairs circulation, which is why half of all those who require leg or foot amputations are diabetics. The restricted circulation also leads to diabetic retinopathy and eventual blindness in many. In fact, diabetes is the primary cause of blindness in those between the ages of twenty and seventy-four. Diabetics also have up to three times the risk of developing a cardiovascular disease and up to four times the risk of suffering from a stroke than those who don't have the disease. Diabetes also increases the risk of periodontal disease, high blood pressure, kidney disease, and nerve damage.

Anyone suffering from diabetes should be under a physician's care. Be sure to let your doctor know if you are taking any herbs, as they will alter your insulin requirement. In addition to the herbs in the following recipes, other helpful herbs include dandelion, goldenseal, juniper berries, and licorice root.

DIABETES TEA #1

30 drops ginseng tincture
60 drops Oregon grape root tincture
1 cup warm water

Combine the above herbs in the warm water in a nonmetallic container; take a third of a cup, up to three times a day.

DIABETES TEA #2

2 teaspoons dried coriander seeds
1 tablespoon ginseng root
2 cups boiling water

Combine the above herbs and cover with the boiling water; steep for 30 minutes; cool and strain. Take half a cup at a time, up to three times daily.

SECRETS
OF NATIVE
AMERICAN
HERBAL
REMEDIES

132

See also CORIANDER; DANDELION; GINSENG; GOLDENSEAL; JUNIPER; LICO-
RICE; *and* OREGON GRAPE *in Part One.*

Diarrhea

Diarrhea is marked by frequent and excessive discharge of watery fecal material. Diarrhea can occur because of bacterial or viral infections or intestinal
parasites. Certain chemicals and drugs can cause diarrhea, as can certain diseases, such as ulcerative colitis and cancer. Emotional stress can also bring
on diarrhea. Food allergies, drinking caffeine or alcohol, or eating unripe
fruit or spoiled food can also bring on an attack.

Excessive or prolonged diarrhea can cause dehydration, which can interfere with the absorption of nutrients. Diarrhea can be especially dangerous in
children because they cannot tolerate much fluid loss.

In addition to the herbs found in the following recipes, other beneficial
herbs to relieve diarrhea include barberry, black currant, Canadian fleabane,
catnip, cayenne, ginger root, marshmallow, mint, pine bark, and witch hazel.

DIARRHEA TEA #1

3 tablespoons agrimony leaves
2 tablespoons self-heal
4 cups water

Combine the herbs in a pan; cover with the water; bring to a boil;
reduce heat and simmer for 30 minutes; cool and strain. Drink as
needed, up to one cup a day.

DIARRHEA TEA #2

2 teaspoons alumroot
2 teaspoons blackberry leaves
2 teaspoons angelica seeds

HEALING
INDIAN
FORMULAS
FOR INDIVIDUAL
CONDITIONS

133

1 teaspoon Oregon grape root

2 cups boiling water

Combine the above herbs in a nonmetallic container. Pour the boiling water over the herbs and steep for 30 minutes; strain; take as needed, up to one cup a day.

IROQUOIS TEA

2 teaspoons raspberry leaves

2 teaspoons strawberry leaves

2 tablespoons yarrow

2 teaspoons yellow dock root

2 cups boiling water

Combine the herbs in a glass container; pour the boiling water over the herbs; steep for 30 minutes; cool and strain. Take up to one cup a day. The Iroquois made a similar tea to treat bloody diarrhea.

See also AGRIMONY; ALUMROOT; ANGELICA; BARBERRY; BLACK CURRANT; BLACKBERRY; CANADIAN FLEABANE; CATNIP; CAYENNE; GINGER; MARSH-MALLOW; PEPPERMINT; PINE; RASPBERRY; SELF-HEAL; STRAWBERRY LEAF; WITCH HAZEL; YARROW; *and* YELLOW DOCK *in Part One*; *and* ALLERGIES; COLITIS; DIARRHEA; *and* STRESS *in Part Two*.

Digestive Problems

(*See* Flatulence; Heartburn; Indigestion)

Dysmenorrhea

Dysmenorrhea means painful menstruation. The pain, which usually begins just before menstruation, may occur in the lower abdomen or the lower back

SECRETS
OF NATIVE
AMERICAN
HERBAL
REMEDIES

134

(and sometimes even into the thighs). Other accompanying symptoms may include nausea, vomiting, headache, and either constipation or diarrhea. This condition affects more than half of all women.

There are two types of dysmenorrhea, primary and secondary. In primary dysmenorrhea, there is no underlying pain causing the disorder. It is thought that the pain occurs when uterine contractions reduce blood supply to the uterus. This may occur if the uterus is in the wrong position, if the cervical opening is narrow, and due to lack of exercise. Secondary dysmenorrhea is when the pain is caused by some gynecological disorder, such as endometriosis (when the endometrium, the tissue that lines the uterus, abnormally grows on surfaces of other structures in the abdominal cavity), adenomyosis (in-growth of the endometrium into the uterine musculature), lesions, inflammation of the fallopian tubes, or uterine fibroids. Uterine fibroids are tumors of the uterus that are not usually cancerous. Also known as myomas, these masses occur in nearly one-quarter of all women by the age of forty. Some women with uterine fibroids may have no symptoms. However, if symptoms are present they include increased frequency of urination, a bloated feeling, pressure, pain, and abnormal bleeding.

In addition to the herbs listed below, other beneficial herbs to help relieve the symptoms of dysmenorrhea and other menstrual disorders include blue vervain, chamomile, elecampane, feverfew, marigold, and peppermint.

DYSMENORRHEA TEA #1

2 teaspoons black haw root or bark
2 teaspoons passionflower
2 cups cold water

Combine the above herbs in a pan and cover with the cold water; soak overnight; strain. Take half a cup, up to four times daily.

DYSMENORRHEA TEA #2

2 teaspoons black cohosh root
1 teaspoon crampbark
1 teaspoon black haw root or bark
1 teaspoon pulsatilla
2 cups water

Combine the above herbs in a pan and cover with the water; bring to a boil and boil for 10 minutes; cool and strain. Take half a cup, up to four times a day.

CRAMP RELIEF TEA

1 teaspoon St. John's wort leaves
1 teaspoon raspberry leaves
1 cup boiling water

Combine the herbs in a glass container and cover with the boiling water; steep for 15 minutes; strain. Drink as needed to relieve cramps.

See also BLACK COHOSH; BLACK HAW; BLUE VERVAIN; CHAMOMILE; CRAMPBARK; ELECAMPANE; FEVERFEW; MARIGOLD; PASSIONFLOWER; PEPPERMINT; PULSATILLA; RASPBERRY; *and* ST. JOHN'S WORT *in Part One.*

Ear Infections

The human ear is composed of the inner ear, the middle ear, and the outer ear. Ear infections can occur in any of the parts of the ear and can spread from one part to another. Usually caused by bacteria or viruses, ear infections can also be caused by trauma. Ear infections are marked by ear pain, fever, reduced hearing ability, and sometimes nausea and vomiting. An outer ear infection

SECRETS
OF NATIVE
AMERICAN
HERBAL
REMEDIES

136

may also be marked by itching and a foul-smelling discharge from the ear. If left unattended, a middle ear infection, also called otitis media, can lead to an inner ear infection. Ear infections can become chronic and cause permanent ear damage.

The following herbs can help build the body's immunity to better fight infection and can also help relieve the discomfort of an ear infection.

EAR INFECTION TEA #1

1 teaspoon echinacea root

1 teaspoon licorice root

2 teaspoons Ginkgo biloba *leaves*

1 teaspoon white willow bark

1 teaspoon grated ginger root

2 cups water

Combine the above herbs in a pan and cover with the water. Bring to a boil and boil for 10 minutes; cool and strain. Take up to one cup a day, a tablespoon at a time.

EAR INFECTION TEA #2

1 teaspoon black cohosh root

1 teaspoon kava kava root

1 teaspoon pulsatilla

2 cups water

Combine the above herbs in a pan and cover with the water. Bring to a boil and boil for 10 minutes; cool and strain. Take two to three tablespoons at a time, up to six times a day.

See BLACK COHOSH; ECHINACEA; GINGER; *GINKGO BILOBA*; KAVA KAVA; LICORICE; PULSATILLA; *and* WHITE WILLOW *in Part One.*

HEALING
INDIAN
FORMULAS
FOR INDIVIDUAL
CONDITIONS

Eczema

Eczema is an inflammatory skin condition also known as dermatitis. Eczema can involve blisters, redness and inflammation, scaling, scabbing, and skin thickening. It also often causes itching that can be quite intense. Although often allergic in nature, eczema can also be caused by an infection or some type of irritation, such as from chemicals. Sometimes eczema occurs when an individual contacts an irritating substance, such as soap, cosmetics, or certain plants and metals.

Dyshidrotic eczema (also called dyshidrosis) is a particular type of eczema marked by small fluid-filled blisters that can appear on the hands and feet. The blisters can be extremely itchy. There is no known cause of dyshidrotic eczema.

ECZEMA TEA

1 teaspoon burdock root
1 teaspoon Oregon grape root
1 teaspoon echinacea root
1 teaspoon yellow dock root
2 cups water

Combine the above herbs in a pan and cover with the water. Bring to a boil; reduce heat and simmer for 10 to 15 minutes; cool and strain. Take a tablespoon at a time, up to half a cup a day.

ECZEMA TOPICAL TEA

1 teaspoon comfrey root
1 teaspoon white oak leaves or bark
1 teaspoon slippery elm bark
2 cups water

SECRETS
OF NATIVE
AMERICAN
HERBAL
REMEDIES

138

Combine the herbs in a container and cover with the water; bring to a boil and boil for 20 to 30 minutes; cool and strain. Use as a topical wash, as needed.

IMMUNITY STRENGTHENER

1 teaspoon echinacea root
1 teaspoon goldenseal root
1 cup boiling water

Combine the herbs in a glass container; cover with the boiling water; steep for 10 to 15 minutes; cool and strain. Take up to one cup a day for no more than seven days.

See also BURDOCK; COMFREY; ECHINACEA; GOLDENSEAL; OREGON GRAPE; SLIPPERY ELM; WHITE OAK; *and* YELLOW DOCK *in Part One.*

Fatigue

Fatigue is more than just being tired. Instead, fatigue is a prolonged or excessive decrease in the ability to function, over and above what normal exertion would cause. Those who push themselves to the point of physical exhaustion are certainly familiar with fatigue. However, fatigue can be a symptom of more than overexertion; it is a symptom of a number of conditions including anemia, circulatory problems (such as angina pectoris, atherosclerosis, and high blood pressure), chronic fatigue syndrome, diabetes, hepatitis, inflammatory bowel disease, multiple sclerosis, and respiratory conditions including pneumonia and pleurisy.

PICK-ME-UP TEA

1 teaspoon Ginkgo biloba *leaves*
1 teaspoon dried mirabilis root

HEALING
INDIAN
FORMULAS
FOR INDIVIDUAL
CONDITIONS

139

1 teaspoon dried ginseng root

1 teaspoon pulsatilla herb

1 teaspoon gotu kola leaves

1 teaspoon St. John's wort leaves

4 cups boiling water

Combine the above herbs in a glass container; cover with the boiling water; steep for 30 minutes; strain. Take as needed.

FATIGUE TEA

1 teaspoon blackberry leaves

1 teaspoon strawberry leaves

1 teaspoon raspberry leaves

2 cups boiling water

Honey

Combine the above herbs in a glass container; cover with the boiling water; steep for 10 minutes; strain. Sweeten with honey if desired. Drink as needed.

See also BLACKBERRY; *GINKGO BILOBA*; GINSENG; GOTU KOLA; MIRABILIS; PULSATILLA; RASPBERRY; ST. JOHN'S WORT; *and* STRAWBERRY LEAF *in Part One; and* ARTEMIA; CHRONIC FATIGUE SYNDROME; CIRCULATORY DISORDERS; COLITIS; DIABETES; LIVER PROBLEMS; MONONUCLEOSIS; PLEURISY; *and* PNEUMONIA *in Part Two.*

Fever

"Normal" body temperature is generally considered to be 98.6°F, although that number may vary between individuals, or even in the same individual at different times of the day. For example, our body temperature is lowest in the early morning and highest in the late afternoon. However, a fever is consid-

SECRETS
OF NATIVE
AMERICAN
HERBAL
REMEDIES

140

ered to be any temperature above 100°F. A fever is usually a sign that the body is fighting off some type of infection.

Whether or not to treat a fever is a very controversial subject. In my opinion, fever is the body's way of repairing itself and should not be suppressed. However, fever in children and in adults with heart illness and other disorders is sometimes serious and may need to be treated.

In addition to the herbs listed below, other beneficial herbs to relieve fever include boneset, cayenne, juniper, marigold, osha root, oxeye daisy, skullcap, and wild indigo root.

FEVER RELIEF TEA #1

1 teaspoon angelica root

1 teaspoon ground ivy leaves

1 teaspoon barberry berries

2 teaspoons peppermint leaves

2 teaspoons blue vervain leaves

1 tablespoon dried yarrow

1 teaspoon catnip leaves

1 cup boiling water

Combine the above herbs. Place one tablespoon of the mixture in a cup; pour the boiling water over the herbs; steep for 30 minutes; strain. Take up to one cup a day.

FEVER RELIEF TEA #2

1 teaspoon echinacea root

1 teaspoon white willow root

1 cup water

Combine the roots in a pan and cover with the water. Bring to a boil; reduce heat and simmer for 30 minutes; cool and strain. Take half a cup, up to four times a day.

See also ANGELICA; BARBERRY; BLUE VERVAIN; CATNIP; ECHINACEA; GROUND IVY; PEPPERMINT; WHITE WILLOW; *and* YARROW *in Part One.*

Flatulence

Flatulence, or gas, is often a symptom of indigestion and can develop when we eat too fast or too much. It can also occur because of allergies or enzyme deficiencies, and is a sign that our bodies are not breaking down the foods that we eat. For example, those people whose bodies do not make the enzyme lactase can't adequately digest the sugars in dairy products. The milk sugars in these products then ferment in the colon, causing gas. High-fiber foods can also cause flatulence, as can beans and cabbage.

ANTI-GAS TEA #1

1 teaspoon dried angelica root

2 teaspoons peppermint leaves

1 teaspoon bee balm leaves

1 cup boiling water

Combine the herbs in a container. Take one tablespoon of the herb mixture and cover with the boiling water; steep for 20 to 30 minutes; strain. Take as needed.

ANTI-GAS TEA #2

2 teaspoons bee balm leaves

2 teaspoons peppermint leaves

2 teaspoons chamomile flowers

1 cup boiling water

Combine the herbs in a container. Take one tablespoon of the mixture and cover with the boiling water; steep for 30 minutes; strain. Take as needed.

SECRETS
OF NATIVE
AMERICAN
HERBAL
REMEDIES

142

ANTI-GAS TEA #3

1 teaspoon catnip leaves
1 teaspoon grated ginger root
2 teaspoons dandelion leaves
2 cups boiling water

Combine the herbs and cover with the boiling water; steep for 20 to 30 minutes; strain. Take as needed.

See also ANGELICA; BEE BALM; CATNIP; CHAMOMILE; DANDELION; GINGER; *and* PEPPERMINT *in Part One.*

Flu

(*See* Influenza)

Gas

(*See* Flatulence)

Gastroesophageal Reflux Disease

(*See* Heartburn)

Gout

Gout is a metabolic disease marked by sudden and severe pain in one or more joints (especially those of the big toe). Gout is caused by excessively high uric acid levels in the blood. This occurs either because the kidneys are not eliminating enough of the body's uric acid or because too much uric acid is being produced.

HEALING
INDIAN
FORMULAS
FOR INDIVIDUAL
CONDITIONS

143

Emotional stress can trigger a gout attack, as can fatigue and minor trauma. Gout also can be caused by renal insufficiency. Gout used to be called "rich man's disease" since an attack can be brought on by consuming a diet rich in fats or alcohol.

In addition to the herbs listed below, other beneficial herbs to relieve the discomfort of gout include barberry, black currant, goldenrod, horehound, horsetail, speedwell, and strawberry.

GOUT TEA #1

4 teaspoons agrimony leaves
2 tablespoons queen of the meadow root
2 cups boiling water

Combine the herbs in a glass container and cover with the boiling water; steep for 30 minutes; cool and strain. Take half a cup, up to four times daily.

GOUT TEA #2

1 teaspoon burdock root
2 tablespoons dandelion leaves
1 cup water

Combine the herbs in a pan and cover with the water. Bring to a boil; remove from the heat; steep for 30 minutes; strain. Take up to one cup per day, a tablespoon at a time.

See also AGRIMONY; BARBERRY; BLACK CURRANT; BURDOCK; DANDELION; GOLDENROD; HOREHOUND; HORSETAIL; QUEEN OF THE MEADOW; SPEEDWELL; *and* STRAWBERRY LEAF *in Part One.*

SECRETS
OF NATIVE
AMERICAN
HERBAL
REMEDIES

144

Hair Loss

Many people experience hair loss as they age, but a number of conditions can also cause hair loss as an unwanted side effect. Some diseases, such as scarlet fever (or other disease marked by high fever), can cause hair loss, as can drug use (especially chemotherapy drugs), and even pregnancy. Sometimes individuals lose their hair for no known reason; however, the tendency toward hair loss is often genetic.

Often topical treatments that bring more blood to the skin can improve hair growth. In fact, many over-the-counter hair products contain cayenne and other irritants for that very reason.

TOPICAL TREATMENT

1 teaspoon cayenne

1 teaspoon yucca root

2 cups water

Combine the herbs in a nonmetallic container and cover with the water; steep for 20 minutes; strain. Apply several times a day, but with caution. Cayenne can increase blood flow to the skin but can also cause blisters if used too often or in too strong a concentration.

See also CAYENNE *and* YUCCA *in Part One.*

Hangover

Everyone knows what a hangover is, even if they have never experienced one firsthand. Excessive alcohol intake dehydrates the body, which is why those suffering from a hangover have a dry mouth and are thirsty. Too much alcohol can also elevate and then drastically drop blood sugar levels, leading to headache, irritability, shakiness or dizziness, and fatigue. Alcohol depletes the body of certain nutrients and can cause fat to build up in the liver. It also causes the stomach to excrete too much acid, which can lead to heartburn, nausea, and vomiting. No wonder a hangover feels so awful.

HANGOVER TEA #1

1 teaspoon ripe barberry berries
1 teaspoon Oregon grape root
2 cups boiling water

Combine the herbs in a nonmetallic container and cover with the boiling water; steep for 30 minutes; cool and strain. Take up to one cup a day, diluted in plenty of cool water.

HANGOVER TEA #2

1 teaspoon bayberry root
1 teaspoon dried goldenseal root
1 teaspoon Oregon grape root
2 cups boiling water

Combine the herbs in a nonmetallic container and cover with the boiling water; steep for 30 minutes; strain. Place a tablespoon of the mixture in an 8-ounce glass of water. Drink several glasses throughout the day.

HANGOVER TEA #3

1 teaspoon catnip leaves
1 teaspoon peppermint leaves
1 teaspoon dried chaparral leaves
2 cups boiling water

Combine the herbs in a nonmetallic container and cover with the boiling water; steep for 20 to 30 minutes; strain. Drink half a cup at a time, up to two cups a day.

SECRETS
OF NATIVE
AMERICAN
HERBAL
REMEDIES

146

See also BARBERRY; BAYBERRY; CATNIP; CHAPARRAL; GOLDENSEAL; ORE-
GON GRAPE; *and* PEPPERMINT *in Part One.*

Hay Fever

(*See* Allergies)

Headache

Headaches are very common and can be dull and steady, stabbing, gnawing,
or throbbing. There are many kinds of headaches with many different causes.
Sometimes tension, fatigue, or stress can cause a headache. Problems with
the eyes, ears, nose, throat, or teeth can bring on a headache, as can allergies,
injuries, infection, tumors, and any number of diseases. Headaches are also
big business. In fact, Americans spend in excess of $1 billion each year buying
medicines to help combat headaches. Most people take nonsteroidal anti-
inflammatory drugs (NSAIDs) such as aspirin, ibuprofen, or indomethacin, or
even stronger painkillers. But these drugs have unwanted, and sometimes
serious, side effects, including ulcers and an increased tendency to bleeding.
Herbs can offer a safer alternative.

In addition to those listed below, other beneficial herbs for headache relief
include chamomile, pleurisy root, willow, and wintergreen.

HEADACHE TEA #1

> *1 teaspoon feverfew leaves*
> *1 teaspoon peppermint leaves*
> *1 cup boiling water*
> *Honey*

Combine the above herbs in a nonmetallic container and cover with
the boiling water; steep for 30 minutes; strain. Add honey to taste.
Take a tablespoon at a time, up to one cup a day.

HEALING
INDIAN
FORMULAS
FOR INDIVIDUAL
CONDITIONS

HEADACHE TEA #2

1 teaspoon catnip leaves
2 teaspoons feverfew leaves
1 to 2 cups boiling water

Combine the catnip and the feverfew in a glass container. Pour one to two cups of boiling water over the herbs; steep for 30 minutes; strain. Take up to one cup a day, a tablespoon at a time.

See also CATNIP; CHAMOMILE; FEVERFEW; PEPPERMINT; PLEURISY ROOT; WHITE WILLOW; *and* WINTERGREEN *in Part One.*

Heartburn

Heartburn is burning stomach pain that can spread up into your throat. Heartburn occurs when hydrochloric acid from your stomach backs up into the esophagus. This condition can result if you gulp your food or drink too much caffeine or alcohol. It can also occur if you eat while stressed or eat certain foods (such as spicy or fatty foods). Antacids are commonly taken for heartburn, but herbs can be just as effective.

In addition to those herbs listed below, other helpful herbs for heartburn include barberry, bayberry, chamomile, chaparral, coriander, dandelion, ginger, hops, Oregon grape, and yellow dock.

Note: If you suffer from heartburn, avoid peppermint. Although it is helpful in treating indigestion and other stomach problems, it can relax the esophageal sphincter and actually increase the tendency toward heartburn.

HEARTBURN TEA #1

1 teaspoon dried angelica root
1 teaspoon crushed juniper berries
1 cup boiling water

SECRETS
OF NATIVE
AMERICAN
HERBAL
REMEDIES

148

Combine the herbs in a nonmetallic container and cover with the boiling water; steep for 20 to 30 minutes; strain. Take a tablespoon at a time, as needed.

HEARTBURN TEA #2

1 teaspoon catnip leaves
1 teaspoon oxeye daisy herb
1 cup boiling water

Combine the herbs in a nonmetallic container and cover with the boiling water; steep for 30 minutes; strain. Take a tablespoon at a time, as needed.

See also ANGELICA; BARBERRY; BAYBERRY; CATNIP; CHAMOMILE; CHAPARRAL; CORIANDER; DANDELION; GINGER; HOPS; JUNIPER; OREGON GRAPE; OXEYE DAISY; *and* YELLOW DOCK *in Part One.*

Hemorrhoids

Once known as "piles," hemorrhoids are enlarged veins of the rectum or anus. Hemorrhoids often protrude and can cause itching and discomfort. Sometimes hemorrhoids bleed, especially during bowel movements. Usually caused by pressure, hemorrhoids most often develop by repeated and excessive straining during bowel movements. Other causes include liver disease, pregnancy, and standing or sitting for long periods of time.

In addition to those herbs listed below, other helpful herbs to relieve the discomfort of hemorrhoids include dandelion, goldenrod, Solomon's seal, wintergreen, and yarrow.

HEALING
INDIAN
FORMULAS
FOR INDIVIDUAL
CONDITIONS

149

HEMORRHOID TEA

1 teaspoon evening primrose
1 teaspoon self-heal
1 teaspoon peppermint leaves
1 quart water

Combine all the ingredients in a pan; bring to a boil and boil until the liquid is reduced to two cups; strain. Drink up to two cups a day.

HEMORRHOID WASH

1 teaspoon blackberry leaves
1 teaspoon witch hazel leaves
1 teaspoon mullein
2 cups boiling water

Combine the herbs in a nonmetallic container and cover with the boiling water; steep for 30 minutes; cool and strain. Use as a wash, whenever needed.

See also BLACKBERRY; DANDELION; EVENING PRIMROSE; GOLDENROD; MULLEIN; PEPPERMINT; SELF-HEAL; SOLOMON'S SEAL; WINTERGREEN; *and* WITCH HAZEL *in Part One*; *and* CONSTIPATION *in Part Two*.

Herpes

(*See* Cold Sores)

SECRETS
OF NATIVE
AMERICAN
HERBAL
REMEDIES

150

Indigestion

Indigestion refers to any gastrointestinal disturbance, such as an upset stomach. Indigestion can occur if you eat too fast, eat too much, eat while emotionally upset, or, for some people, eat the wrong foods. Caffeine, high-fiber foods, alcohol, and carbonated drinks are often indigestion culprits. Sometimes allergies can cause indigestion. Indigestion can be a symptom of a number of diseases, including pancreatitis, ulcers, gastritis, and cholecystis. Often, however, there is no known cause for indigestion.

A number of herbs can improve digestion and relieve the distress caused by indigestion. In addition to those listed below, other helpful herbs include barberry, bayberry, catnip, echinacea, and Oregon grape.

INDIGESTION TEA #1

1 teaspoon blue cohosh root
1 teaspoon coneflower root
1 cup boiling water

Combine the above herbs in a glass container. Pour the boiling water over the herbs; steep for 30 minutes; cool and strain. Take as needed, up to one cup a day.

INDIGESTION TEA #2

1 teaspoon angelica root
1 teaspoon grated ginger root
2 teaspoons chamomile flowers
2 teaspoons peppermint leaves
1 cup boiling water

Combine the above ingredients in a container. Take one tablespoon of the herb mixture and place in the boiling water; steep for 30 minutes; cool and strain. Take as needed, up to two cups a day.

INDIGESTION TEA #3

1 teaspoon licorice root
1 teaspoon peppermint leaves
2 cups boiling water

Combine the above herbs in a nonmetallic container and cover with the boiling water; steep for 15 to 20 minutes; strain. Take as needed, up to one cup a day.

See also ANGELICA; BARBERRY; BAYBERRY; BLUE COHOSH; CATNIP; CHAMOMILE; CONEFLOWER; ECHINACEA; GINGER; LICORICE; OREGON GRAPE; *and* PEPPERMINT *in Part One.*

Influenza

Often called "flu" or "grippe," influenza is an infectious viral disease that causes fever, headache, chills, loss of appetite, weakness, and general pains and aches. The mucous membranes of the throat and nose may also be inflamed. Note that, although many people refer to stomach upset as the "flu," influenza is not the cause of intestinal upsets. Influenza spreads rapidly and is partly transmitted by coughing and sneezing. The flu virus weakens the body's defenses against bacteria. This is why individuals suffering from the flu risk developing pneumonia (either from the virus itself or from a secondary bacterial infection). The elderly and those whose health is already compromised with an underlying health problem (such as a cardiovascular disease) are at increased risk of developing complications. Usually, however, influenza lasts only a few days.

There is no cure for the flu. However, herbs can help relieve the uncomfortable symptoms of influenza.

SECRETS
OF NATIVE
AMERICAN
HERBAL
REMEDIES

152

INFLUENZA TEA #1

2 teaspoons bayberry bark
2 teaspoons grated ginger root
1 teaspoon powdered cayenne
2 cups boiling water
Honey

Combine the above herbs. Place one teaspoon of the mixture in a glass container and cover with the boiling water; steep for 30 minutes; cool and strain. Add honey to taste. Take a tablespoonful at a time throughout the day.

INFLUENZA TEA #2

2 teaspoons black cohosh root
2 teaspoons powdered Indian root
2 teaspoons chamomile flower
2 cups water
Honey

Place the above herbs in a pan; cover with the water. Bring to a boil; reduce heat and simmer for 30 minutes. Add honey to taste. Take one tablespoon in two cups of water, several times a day.

See also BAYBERRY; BLACK COHOSH; CAYENNE; CHAMOMILE; GINGER; *and* INDIAN ROOT *in Part One.*

Insomnia

Insomnia is any difficulty in sleeping. Some people find it difficult to fall asleep, while others can fall asleep easily but don't stay asleep. Nearly one-fourth of all Americans have an occasional problem sleeping, but some people (as much as 10 percent of the American population) suffer from chronic insomnia. Insomnia can occur for a number of reasons, including stress and nervous tension, excessive intake of caffeinated drinks, and irregular sleeping habits.

Insomnia can lead to fatigue and an inability to function at an optimal energy level during the day. Irritability, daytime drowsiness, and memory impairment often affect those suffering from insomnia.

INSOMNIA RELIEF TEA #1

1 teaspoon chamomile flowers
1 teaspoon hops
1 teaspoon valerian root
1 cup boiling water

Combine the above herbs. Take one tablespoon of the mixture and cover with the boiling water; let steep for 30 minutes; strain. Drink warm, as needed, half a cup at a time.

INSOMNIA RELIEF TEA #2

2 teaspoons catnip leaves
1 teaspoon hops
2 teaspoons chamomile flower
2 teaspoons passionflower
1 cup boiling water

Combine the above herbs in a glass container; cover with the boiling water; steep for 30 minutes; cool and strain. Take as needed for insomnia.

See also CATNIP; CHAMOMILE; HOPS; PASSIONFLOWER; *and* VALERIAN *in Part One.*

SECRETS
OF NATIVE
AMERICAN
HERBAL
REMEDIES

154

Intestinal Worms

A number of worms infest humans, including hookworms, threadworms, pinworms, tapeworms, whipworms, and flukes. Symptoms can include abdominal pain, diarrhea, anemia, weight loss, respiratory symptoms, and itching.

Proper sanitation, including good personal hygiene, adequate toilet facilities, and clean water and soil, go a long way in preventing worm infestations. Herbs have been used for thousands of years to treat worms. In addition to those herbs listed below, other herbs traditionally used to eliminate worms include agrimony, black currants, blue vervain, catnip, elecampane, ginseng, hops, juniper, lady's slipper, nettle, and pipsissewa.

INTESTINAL WORM TEA #1

1 teaspoon mirabilis root
1 teaspoon echinacea root
2 cups water

Combine the above herbs in a pan and cover with the water; bring to a boil and boil for 15 to 20 minutes; cool and strain. Take half a cup every night at bedtime, for three to four nights.

INTESTINAL WORM TEA #2

1 teaspoon blue cohosh root
1 teaspoon feverfew leaves
1 teaspoon Canadian fleabane leaves
1 teaspoon horehound leaves
2 cups boiling water

Combine the above herbs in a nonmetallic container and cover with the boiling water; steep for 30 minutes; cool and strain. Take half a cup for four nights in a row.

See also AGRIMONY; BLACK CURRANT; BLUE COHOSH; BLUE VERVAIN; CANADIAN FLEABANE; CATNIP; ECHINACEA; ELECAMPANE; FEVERFEW; GINSENG; HOPS; HOREHOUND; JUNIPER; LADY'S SLIPPER; MIRABILIS; NETTLE; *and* PIPSISSEWA *in Part One.*

Kidney and Bladder Problems

The kidneys and the bladder play important roles in the body. The main function of the kidneys is to remove excess fluid and waste products from the body through the urine. They also regulate the body's potassium and sodium levels, as well as its pH balance, and produce hormones that affect other organs, including erythropoietin (which stimulates red blood cell production) and renin (which helps blood flow). Since the kidneys are such a vital body organ, any injury or disease that interferes with kidney function has the potential to be very serious. Kidney disease is actually a catch-all term that includes diseases ranging from kidney stones and urinary tract infections to more serious disorders such as glomerulonephritis and polycystic kidney disease. Although each kidney condition has its own unique characteristics, certain symptoms are associated with the majority of kidney problems. These include a frequent urge to urinate, chills, fluid retention (puffiness in the face and limbs or resulting weight gain), back pain (felt just under the ribs), vomiting, fever, pain, nausea, loss of appetite, and a burning sensation during urination. The urine may be cloudy or bloody. Both kidneys are usually affected by any kidney disease. If the ability of the kidneys to filter blood is seriously damaged, excess fluid and wastes may build up in the body. This causes symptoms of kidney failure and severe swelling.

The bladder is a hollow organ with muscular walls that is part of the urinary tract. Urine continuously drains into the bladder from the kidney. In an adult, the bladder can hold about two cups of urine. As the bladder fills, it causes discomfort and, hence, the urge to urinate.

Bladder infections and inflammation can occur in any area of the bladder

SECRETS
OF NATIVE
AMERICAN
HERBAL
REMEDIES

156

and servicing tissue. The most common bladder disorder, cystitis, is an infection or inflammation of the bladder. Symptoms of cystitis include a frequent urge to urinate (even though the bladder may be empty), excessive night urination, and dark or cloudy urine with an unpleasant or strong odor. Lower abdominal pain and a painful, burning sensation on urination may accompany the infection. There may be blood in the urine, and you may suffer chills, fever, loss of appetite, nausea, vomiting, and back pain.

In addition to the herbs listed below, other beneficial herbs include barberry, bilberry, horsetail, marshmallow, sarsaparilla, and speedwell.

KIDNEY TEA

1 teaspoon Oregon grape root
1 teaspoon wild cherry root
2 cups water

Place the above herbs in a pan and cover with the water; bring the mixture to a boil; reduce heat and simmer for 30 minutes; cool and strain. Place a tablespoon of the resulting tea in an 8-ounce glass of water and stir well. Drink one to two tablespoons at a time, up to one cup a day.

TO IMPROVE URINE FLOW

1 teaspoon horseradish root
1 teaspoon queen of the meadow
1 teaspoon parsley
1 cup boiling water

Combine the above herbs and cover with the boiling water; steep for 30 minutes; strain. Take one tablespoon of the mixture in a glass of apple juice, three or four times daily.

BLADDER TEA #1

1 teaspoon black currants

1 teaspoon pipsissewa

1 cup boiling water

Combine the above herbs and cover with the boiling water; steep for 15 minutes; strain. Use two to three times daily for inflammation of the bladder, up to three cups a day, for no more than three days.

BLADDER TEA #2

1 teaspoon uva ursi leaves and stems

1 teaspoon Oregon grape

2 cups water

Place the herbs in a pan and cover with the water. Bring to a boil and boil for 30 minutes; strain. Take as needed.

See also BLACK CURRANT; HORSERADISH; OREGON GRAPE; PARSLEY; PIP-SISSEWA; QUEEN OF THE MEADOW; UVA URSI; *and* WILD CHERRY *in Part One.*

Laryngitis

Laryngitis is inflammation of the larynx—your "voice box." If you have laryngitis, you have lost your voice. It can result from a viral or a bacterial infection. Laryngitis may also occur during bronchitis, influenza, measles, pneumonia, and whooping cough, or because of overuse of the voice or exposure to allergies. The infection or irritation causes the vocal cords to swell, resulting in hoarseness and loss of voice.

SECRETS
OF NATIVE
AMERICAN
HERBAL
REMEDIES

158

LARYNGITIS TEA

1 teaspoon coltsfoot leaves

1 tablespoon marshmallow leaves

1 teaspoon licorice root

1 teaspoon mullein leaves

1 cup boiling water

Combine the above herbs. Take two teaspoons of the mixture and cover with the boiling water; steep for 30 minutes; strain. Sweeten, if desired. Take as needed, a tablespoon or two at a time.

See also COLTSFOOT; LICORICE; MARSHMALLOW; *and* MULLEIN *in Part One*; *and* BRONCHITIS; COUGHS AND COLDS; CROUP; INFLUENZA; MEASLES; PNEUMONIA; SORE THROAT; *and* TONSILLITIS *in Part Two*.

Liver Problems

The liver is the largest organ in the body. It has a number of jobs, including forming and excreting bile, controlling cholesterol metabolism, metabolizing drugs and other substances, and forming urea, albumin, enzymes, and other proteins. The most common disorders affecting the liver include hepatitis and cirrhosis.

Hepatitis is an inflammation of the liver, which is marked by tenderness and swelling, mild fever, fatigue, joint or muscle aches, vomiting, nausea, loss of appetite, and possibly diarrhea. Many cases go undiagnosed, since these symptoms are indicative of so many other conditions, including the stomach flu.

According to the American Liver Foundation, viral hepatitis is the most common of the serious contagious viral diseases that attack the liver. Although hepatitis can be caused by a virus, it also may be caused by drugs, alcohol, and

HEALING
INDIAN
FORMULAS
FOR INDIVIDUAL
CONDITIONS

159

chemicals. Of the viral-caused forms, there are at least five types of hepatitis presently known: Hepatitis A, B, C, D, and E. Rarer causes include other viruses (such as yellow fever, leptospirosis, cytomegalovirus, and infectious mononucleosis). Hepatitis can cause permanent damage to the liver.

Cirrhosis is a chronic liver disease. In the United States, most cases of cirrhosis are due to chronic alcoholism; however, it can also be caused by severe reactions to prescription drugs, biliary obstruction, prolonged exposure to environmental toxins, and abnormal storage of metals by the body.

Cirrhosis is marked by destruction of normal liver tissue. This destruction leads to scar formation, which interferes with normal liver function. Unfortunately, in many cases, obvious symptoms do not occur until the disease is quite advanced.

In addition to those herbs listed below, other beneficial herbs for liver disorders include blue vervain, devil's claw, elecampane, horseradish, hyssop, oxeye daisy, peppermint, and yarrow.

LIVER TEA #1

1 teaspoon blue flag

1 teaspoon Oregon grape root

1 teaspoon dandelion

1 teaspoon redroot

3 teaspoons milk thistle

1 teaspoon yellow dock root

1 teaspoon ocotillo bark

1 cup boiling water

Combine the above herbs in a container. Take one tablespoon of the mixture and cover with the boiling water; steep for 30 minutes; cool and strain. Take up to one cup per day, as needed.

SECRETS
OF NATIVE
AMERICAN
HERBAL
REMEDIES

160

LIVER TEA #2

2 teaspoons chicory flowers
4 teaspoons speedwell
4 teaspoons dandelion root
1 cup boiling water

Combine the above herbs in a glass container. Take two teaspoons of the mixture and cover with the boiling water; steep for 30 minutes; strain. Take a tablespoon at a time, up to one cup a day.

LIVER TEA #3

1 teaspoon chaparral leaves
2 teaspoons milk thistle seed
1 teaspoon burdock root
2 teaspoons Oregon grape root
1 teaspoon echinacea
1 teaspoon yellow dock
1 cup boiling water

Combine the above herbs in a container. Take two teaspoons of the mixture and cover with the boiling water; steep for 30 minutes; strain. Take up to one cup per day, as needed.

LIVER TEA #4

1 teaspoon milk thistle tincture
40 drops bayberry tincture
1 cup warm water

Combine all ingredients. Take one-fourth of the mixture four times daily.

See also BLUE FLAG; BLUE VERVAIN; BURDOCK; CHAPARRAL; CHICORY; DANDELION; DEVIL'S CLAW; ECHINACEA; ELECAMPANE; HORSERADISH, HYSSOP; MILK THISTLE; OCOTILLO BARK; OREGON GRAPE; OXEYE DAISY; PEPPERMINT; REDROOT; SPEEDWELL; YARROW; *and* YELLOW DOCK *in Part One.*

Macular Degeneration

The macula is part of the retina. As we age, the arteries of the eye begin to harden. This can result in decreased blood flow to the eye and, ultimately, blockage of the small arteries. This, in turn, causes the macula to degenerate. The resulting condition is called macular degeneration. It is the leading cause of disturbed vision in the elderly and affects nearly 35 percent of all individuals by the time they reach seventy-five years of age.

A visual distortion in one eye may be the first symptom of macular degeneration, which can occur slowly or come on suddenly. This condition is marked by blurred, or even totally absent, central vision.

MACULAR TEA

1 teaspoon bilberry
1 teaspoon pulsatilla
1 teaspoon black currants
1 teaspoon raspberry leaves
2 cups boiling water

Combine the above herbs and cover with the boiling water; steep for 20 to 30 minutes; strain and drink, as needed, up to two cups per day.

CIRCULATION TEA

1 teaspoon black cohosh root
2 teaspoons Ginkgo biloba
1 cup boiling water

SECRETS
OF NATIVE
AMERICAN
HERBAL
REMEDIES

162

Combine the above herbs and cover with the boiling water; steep for 20 to 30 minutes; strain. Take up to one cup per day, a tablespoon at a time.

See also BILBERRY; BLACK COHOSH; BLACK CURRANT; *GINKGO BILOBA*; PULSATILLA; *and* RASPBERRY *in Part One.*

Malaise

Sometimes we may feel a little under the weather for no apparent reason. There may be no specific symptoms, just a general feeling of illness. This is called malaise. When you experience this feeling, try the following recipes.

GENERAL ILLNESS TONIC

1 teaspoon wild cherry bark
1 teaspoon red willow bark
1 teaspoon wild cherry root
1 teaspoon red willow root
4 cups water

Combine the herbs in a pan and cover with the water. Bring to a boil and boil for 30 minutes; strain and cool. Refrigerate. Take one to two tablespoons at a time, as needed. The Okanagan-Colville Indians drank this decoction for any type of sickness.

ILLNESS PREVENTATIVE

1 teaspoon bayberry root
1 teaspoon Indian root
4 teaspoons echinacea
1 teaspoon ocotillo bark
2 teaspoons goldenseal
1 teaspoon redroot
4 cups water

Combine the herbs in a pan and cover with the water. Bring to a boil and boil for 30 minutes; strain and cool. Refrigerate. Take one to two tablespoons daily.

ROOT TONIC

1 teaspoon black cohosh root

1 teaspoon elecampane root

1 teaspoon stone root

2 cups water

Combine the herbs in a pan and cover with water. Bring to a boil and boil for 30 minutes; strain. Drink up to one cup a day. This tea may be refrigerated and consumed either warm or cold.

See also BAYBERRY; ECHINACEA; GOLDENSEAL; INDIAN ROOT; OCOTILLO BARK; RED WILLOW; REDROOT; *and* WILD CHERRY *in Part One.*

Measles

Measles is a highly contagious acute viral disease. This disease is marked by a characteristic rash, fever, sneezing, coughing, and lymph node tenderness. Spread primarily by airborne droplets that travel from the throat, mouth, or nose of an infected person, there are two types of measles, rubella and rubeola. German (or three-day) measles is actually *rubella.* The second kind, rubeola, is sometimes called the seven-day measles. Most people have had the disease as children and have developed an immunity or have been immunized against it.

Although measles is fairly well controlled in the United States because of vaccinations, it continues to be a major killer throughout the rest of the world, responsible for over one million deaths every year.

Children with measles should be under the care of a qualified health-care practitioner.

SECRETS
OF NATIVE
AMERICAN
HERBAL
REMEDIES

164

MEASLES TEA #1

1 teaspoon goldenseal root
1 teaspoon marshmallow root
1 cup boiling water

Combine the above herbs in a nonmetallic container and cover with the boiling water; steep for 30 minutes; cool and strain. Take up to one cup a day, a tablespoon or two at a time.

MEASLES TEA #2

2 teaspoons echinacea root
3 teaspoons pau d'arco bark
1 teaspoon mullein leaves
3 teaspoons yellow dock root
1 cup boiling water

Combine the above herbs in a container. Take one teaspoon of the mixture and cover with the boiling water; steep for 20 minutes; strain. Take up to two cups a day, a tablespoon or two at a time.

See also ECHINACEA; GOLDENSEAL; MARSHMALLOW; MULLEIN; PAU D'ARCO; *and* YELLOW DOCK *in Part One.*

Menstrual Cramps

(*See* Dysmenorrhea)

Migraines

(*See* Headaches)

HEALING
INDIAN
FORMULAS
FOR INDIVIDUAL
CONDITIONS

165

Mononucleosis

Mononucleosis (mono) is a mildly infectious disease caused by the Epstein-Barr virus (EBV) and cytomegalovirus (CMV). Marked by severe fatigue, fever, sore throat, swollen lymph glands, loss of appetite, muscle aches and pain, and a general ill feeling, mono can also lead to an enlarged spleen and jaundice. Also called "kissing" disease (because it can be spread in this way), mono can occur at any time during life. This illness lasts about two weeks, but it may be several more weeks before fatigue diminishes and your normal energy levels return.

MONO TEA #1

1 teaspoon burdock root

1 teaspoon ginseng root

1 teaspoon cayenne

1 teaspoon goldenseal root

2 cups water

Place the above herbs in a pan and cover with the water. Bring to a boil and boil until reduced by half. Cool and strain. Take up to one cup a day, a tablespoon or two at a time.

MONO TEA #2

2 teaspoons echinacea root

3 teaspoons pau d'arco bark

1 teaspoon mullein leaves

3 teaspoons yellow dock root

1 cup boiling water

Combine the above herbs in a container. Take one teaspoon of the mixture and cover with the boiling water; steep for 20 minutes; strain. Take up to two cups a day, a tablespoon or two at a time.

SECRETS
OF NATIVE
AMERICAN
HERBAL
REMEDIES

166

See also Burdock; Cayenne; Echinacea; Ginseng; Goldenseal; Mullein; Pau d'Arco; *and* Yellow Dock *in Part One.*

Mumps

Mumps is a mildly contagious viral infection that causes pain and swelling of the salivary glands. Mumps is marked by face pain and neck swelling. Other symptoms include fever, sore throat, headache, chills, and aches. Mumps is only spread by contact with infected saliva. Signs and symptoms of mumps may not appear until two to three or more weeks after infection.

Children are most usually affected by mumps, although vaccinations have reduced the incidence of mumps in children, at least within the United States. Children with mumps should be under the care of a qualified health-care practitioner. When mumps affects older individuals, the testes, pancreas, prostate, and central nervous system also may become involved.

MUMPS TEA #1

20 drops black cohosh tincture
30 drops echinacea tincture
1 cup warm water

Combine the above tinctures with the warm water. Take one-third cup, up to three times daily.

MUMPS TEA #2

1 teaspoon echinacea root
1 teaspoon mullein leaves
1 teaspoon goldenseal root
1 teaspoon yellow dock root
1 cup boiling water

HEALING
INDIAN
FORMULAS
FOR INDIVIDUAL
CONDITIONS

167

Combine the above herbs in a container. Take one teaspoon of the mixture and cover with the boiling water; steep for 20 minutes; strain. Take up two cups a day, a tablespoon or two at a time.

See also BLACK COHOSH; ECHINACEA; GOLDENSEAL; MULLEIN; *and* YELLOW DOCK *in Part One.*

Nausea and Vomiting

Nausea is an unpleasant feeling that you are about to vomit. It is often accompanied by excess salivation and sometimes stomach cramping. A number of diseases and conditions can cause nausea, including food poisoning (and other bacterial infections), viral infections, overeating or overdrinking, gallstones, pancreatitis, and cancer. It can also occur because of motion sickness, headache, or pregnancy. Sometimes unpleasant smells or tastes, and even emotional anxiety, can bring on nausea.

In addition to those herbs listed below, other beneficial herbs to relieve nausea include bayberry, bee balm, chaparral, horehound, and Oregon grape.

NAUSEA TEA #1

> *1 teaspoon grated ginger root*
> *1 teaspoon yerba mansa root*
> *1 teaspoon peppermint leaves*
> *2 cups boiling water*

Combine the above herbs in a nonmetallic container and cover with the boiling water; steep for 30 minutes; cool and strain. Take as needed, a tablespoon at a time, up to two cups a day.

NAUSEA TEA #2

> *1 teaspoon catnip leaves*
> *1 teaspoon chamomile flowers*
> *1 cup boiling water*

SECRETS
OF NATIVE
AMERICAN
HERBAL
REMEDIES

168

Combine the above ingredients in a nonmetallic container and cover with the boiling water; steep for 20 to 30 minutes; cool and strain. Take as needed.

See also BAYBERRY; BEE BALM; CATNIP; CHAMOMILE; CHAPARRAL; GINGER; HOREHOUND; OREGON GRAPE; PEPPERMINT; *and* YERBA MANSA *in Part One.*

Nervousness

We've all been nervous at one time or another. Shaking hands, a trembling voice, and a rolling stomach are some of the most common symptoms of nervousness. A number of situations can bring on nervousness, including public speaking.

In addition to those herbs listed below, other helpful herbs to combat nervousness include blue vervain, chamomile, passionflower, and pulsatilla.

NERVE TEA #1

1 teaspoon betony leaves
1 teaspoon kava kava root
1 teaspoon hops
1 teaspoon dried skullcap
1 cup boiling water

Combine the above herbs. Take one tablespoon of the mixture and cover with the boiling water; steep for 30 minutes; cool and strain. Take one tablespoon at a time, as needed, up to one cup a day.

NERVE TEA #2

1 teaspoon powdered ginger
1 teaspoon powdered valerian root
1 teaspoon powdered pleurisy root
2 cups boiling water

HEALING
INDIAN
FORMULAS
FOR INDIVIDUAL
CONDITIONS

169

Combine the above herbs and cover with the boiling water; steep for 30 minutes; cool and strain. Take one tablespoon at a time, as needed, up to two cups a day.

NERVE TEA #3

1 to 2 teaspoons peppermint leaves
1 teaspoon valerian root
2 cups boiling water

Combine the above herbs and cover with the boiling water; steep for 20 to 30 minutes; strain. Drink up to one cup per day, as needed.

See also BETONY; BLUE VERVAIN; CHAMOMILE; GINGER; HOPS; KAVA KAVA; PASSIONFLOWER; PEPPERMINT; PLEURISY ROOT; PULSATILLA; SKULLCAP; *and* VALERIAN *in Part One.*

Obesity

According to most authorities, you are obese if you weigh 20 percent or more above what is considered "normal" weight for your height, build, age, and sex. According to one report, more than one-third of all Americans are now obese. In fact, more than 58 million Americans are now considered obese.

Being obese makes an individual more susceptible to atherosclerosis, diabetes, elevated cholesterol, glandular dysfunction, heart disease, high blood pressure, and hypoglycemia. Statistics prove that those who are not obese live longer and healthier lives.

Obesity can occur for a variety of reasons, although excessive food intake and insufficient exercise are often the culprits. Other reasons for obesity include hormonal disorders, certain drugs (such as corticosteroids), psychological factors, and metabolic disorders. Once any underlying physiological

SECRETS
OF NATIVE
AMERICAN
HERBAL
REMEDIES

170

reason is identified and treated, most experts agree that, to lose weight, it is important to eat less and exercise more.

OBESITY TEA

1 tablespoon dandelion leaves
1 teaspoon mirabilis root
2 cups boiling water

Combine the above herbs and cover with the boiling water; steep for 30 minutes; cool and strain. Take half a cup before every meal.

See also DANDELION AND MIRABILIS *in Part One.*

Pleurisy

Pleurisy is an inflammation of the pleura (the double membrane that covers each lung and lines the chest cavity). This condition is marked by sudden chest pain that may be minor or intense and stabbing. Fever may also be present. There may also be coughing, breathing may be shallow, and there may be a general ill feeling. Pleurisy can occur because of an injury or irritation to the pleura or because of a viral or bacterial infection. It can also be a complication of tuberculosis, cancer, pneumonia, or some other condition.

In addition to those herbs listed below, other helpful herbs include echinacea, ginger, *Ginkgo biloba,* licorice, and white willow.

PLEURISY TEA #1

2 teaspoons boneset
3 teaspoons licorice root
2 teaspoon elder flowers
4 teaspoons pleurisy root
3 cups water

HEALING
INDIAN
FORMULAS
FOR INDIVIDUAL
CONDITIONS

171

Combine the above herbs in a pan and cover with the water; bring to a boil; reduce heat; simmer for 10 minutes; strain. Take up to one cup a day, a tablespoon at a time.

PLEURISY TEA #2

2 chamomile flowers
3 nettle leaves
3 coltsfoot leaves
1 cup boiling water

Combine the above herbs in a container. Take two teaspoons of the mixture and cover with the boiling water; steep for 30 minutes; strain. Take up to two cups a day, a tablespoon at a time.

See also BLACK ELDER; BONESET; CHAMOMILE; ECHINACEA; GINGER; GINKGO BILOBA; LICORICE; NETTLE; PLEURISY BOOT; *and* WHITE WILLOW *in Part One; and* COUGHS AND COLDS; CROUP; PNEUMONIA; *and* TUBERCULOSIS *in Part Two.*

Pneumonia

Pneumonia is an acute lung infection that can be caused by viruses or bacteria. Inhaling toxic chemicals can also bring on the disease in some individuals. Symptoms of pneumonia include chest pain, difficulty breathing, and coughing. There may also be chills followed by a fever. Sometimes nausea and vomiting may occur. Every year, nearly 2 million Americans get pneumonia and nearly 70,000 of those die.

In addition to those herbs listed in the formulas below, other beneficial herbs include agrimony, black cohosh, chamomile, goldenseal, osha root, pleurisy root, redroot, and wild cherry.

SECRETS
OF NATIVE
AMERICAN
HERBAL
REMEDIES

172

PNEUMONIA TEA #1

1 teaspoon catnip leaves
1 teaspoon peppermint leaves
1 cup boiling water

Combine the above herbs in a nonmetallic container and cover with the boiling water; steep for 30 minutes; strain. Take warm, as needed, up to two cups a day.

PNEUMONIA TEA #2

1 teaspoon coltsfoot leaves
1 teaspoon horehound leaves
1 teaspoon elderflowers
1 teaspoon marshmallow root
1 teaspoon ground ivy
4 cups boiling water

Combine the above herbs in a nonmetallic container and cover with the boiling water; steep for 30 minutes; strain. Take warm, a tablespoon at a time, up to one cup per day.

See also AGRIMONY; BLACK COHOSH; BLACK ELDER; CATNIP; CHAMOMILE; COLTSFOOT; GOLDENSEAL; GROUND IVY; HOREHOUND; MARSHMALLOW; OSHA ROOT; PEPPERMINT; PLEURISY ROOT; REDROOT; *and* WILD CHERRY *in Part One.*

Premenstrual Syndrome

Premenstrual syndrome (PMS) appears to be a hormonal disorder that occurs one to two weeks before monthly menstruation begins. PMS is marked by a

HEALING
INDIAN
FORMULAS
FOR INDIVIDUAL
CONDITIONS

173

myriad of digestive, emotional, and physical symptoms. These symptoms include diarrhea (and sometimes constipation), abdominal bloating, anxiety, panic attacks, mood swings, nervousness, depression, irritability, hostility, mental confusion, difficulty concentrating, breast tenderness and swelling, fluid retention, headache, weight gain, joint pain, muscle spasms, fatigue, and sometimes food cravings.

PMS affects approximately 40 percent of all women. The symptoms of almost 10 percent of PMS sufferers are so severe as to interfere with their business and personal lives. The causes of PMS are varied, although estrogen and prostaglandins are usually involved. Estrogen levels alter during the days before the onset of menstruation. This can cause an increase in body fluids, which, in turn, leads to the typical symptoms of weight gain, bloating, and edema. Prostaglandin levels also increase during PMS, which can bring on several of the characteristic symptoms. Prostaglandins are hormonelike chemicals involved in inflammation.

PMS TEA #1

1 teaspoon cornsilk
1 teaspoon pulsatilla
6 teaspoons crampbark
1 teaspoon raspberry leaf
1 teaspoon ocotillo bark
1 cup boiling water

Combine the above herbs. Take two teaspoons of the mixture and cover with the boiling water; steep for 30 minutes; strain. Take as needed throughout the day, up to one cup per day.

PMS TEA #2

1 teaspoon black cohosh root
1 teaspoon passionflower
1 teaspoon Oregon grape root

SECRETS
OF NATIVE
AMERICAN
HERBAL
REMEDIES

174

1 teaspoon white willow bark

2 cups water

Place the above herbs in a pan and cover with the water. Bring to a boil and boil for 20 minutes; cool and strain. Take one to two tablespoons at a time, up to one cup per day as needed.

PMS TEA #3

1 teaspoon black haw

1 teaspoon licorice root

1 teaspoon evening primrose

1 teaspoon milk thistle

3 cups boiling water

Combine the above herbs in a nonmetallic container and cover with the boiling water; steep for 20 to 35 minutes; strain. Take half a cup, four times a day.

See also BLACK COHOSH; BLACK HAW; CORNSILK; CRAMPBARK; EVENING PRIMROSE; LICORICE; MILK THISTLE; OCOTILLO BARK; OREGON GRAPE; PASSIONFLOWER; PULSATILLA; *and* WHITE WILLOW *in Part One.*

Prostate Problems

The prostate is a chestnut-sized male gland through which both urine and sperm pass. For unknown reasons, the prostate gradually enlarges as men age. In fact, 60 percent of all men over the age of fifty have an enlarged prostate. As the prostate enlarges, it presses on the neck of the bladder and interferes with the excretion of urine. This can weaken and strain the bladder and may lead to kidney infection.

The most common prostate disorders are enlargement of the prostate (benign prostate hyperplasia), prostatitis (inflammation of the prostate gland),

and prostate cancer. Symptoms of prostate disorders include a frequent urge to urinate, difficulty starting urination and emptying the bladder, groin pain, and lower back pain. There may also be chills and fever, muscle and joint aches, and burning (or bleeding) with urination.

In addition to those herbs listed below, other beneficial herbs include black cohosh, goldenrod, horsetail, kava kava, nettle, white cedar, and yerba mansa.

PROSTATE TEA #1

1 teaspoon goldenseal root
1 teaspoon fringe tree bark
4 teaspoons saw palmetto berries
2 cups boiling water

Combine the above herbs in a nonmetallic container and cover with the boiling water; steep for 30 minutes; strain. Take up to one cup per day.

PROSTATE TEA #2

1 teaspoon couch grass rhizome
1 teaspoon juniper berries
2 cups boiling water

Combine the above herbs and cover with the boiling water; steep for 10 minutes. Take a quarter cup, five times daily.

See also BLACK COHOSH; COUCH GRASS; GOLDENROD; GOLDENSEAL; HORSE-TAIL; JUNIPER; KAVA KAVA; NETTLE; SAW PALMETTO; WHITE CEDAR LEAF TIPS; *and* YERBA MANSA *in Part One.*

SECRETS
OF NATIVE
AMERICAN
HERBAL
REMEDIES

176

Psoriasis

Psoriasis is a skin disease marked by red, itchy patches of various sizes. The patches are usually well defined, dry, and may be covered with loose, silvery scales. The skin may burn, itch, and bleed easily. Although lesions can occur anywhere on the body, they most often are found on the elbows, wrists, forearms, legs, knees, ankles, and scalp. They can also appear on the soles of the feet, and on the abdomen, chest, and back. The fingernails and toenails can develop ridges and pits, losing their luster.

Psoriasis can be mild, moderate, or severe and disabling. It may go away, but it always comes back (psoriasis is a chronic and recurrent disease). Usually, psoriasis requires ongoing treatment to achieve periods of clear skin, maintain health, and restore function. At present, there is no universally effective therapy.

Psoriasis is not communicable—you can't catch it from someone who has it. However, it does seems to run in families. But having someone in the family with the disease does not guarantee you will also suffer, since studies show that nearly one-third of those who are genetically predisposed to psoriasis never develop it. Certain factors may trigger psoriasis, such as injury to the skin, certain drugs (such as lithium), stress, cold weather, staphylococcus or streptococcus bacterial infections, surgery, or sunburn. However, a certain amount of solar radiation also can lead to symptom improvement.

PSORIASIS TEA #1

1 teaspoon barberry
1 teaspoon burdock root
2 cups boiling water

Combine the above herbs in a nonmetallic container and cover with the boiling water; steep for 20 to 30 minutes; strain. Drink a tablespoon at a time, up to one cup a day.

HEALING
INDIAN
FORMULAS
FOR INDIVIDUAL
CONDITIONS

177

PSORIASIS TEA #2

1 teaspoon ocotillo bark
1 teaspoon yellow dock root
1 teaspoon Oregon grape root
3 cups water

Combine the above herbs in a pan and cover with the water; bring to a boil and simmer until the liquid is reduced by half. Cool and strain. Take a tablespoon at a time, several times a day.

TOPICAL TEA

1 teaspoon comfrey root
1 teaspoon white oak leaves or bark
1 teaspoon slippery elm bark
2 cups water

Place the herbs in a container in a nonmetallic container and cover with the water; bring to a boil and boil for 20 to 30 minutes; cool and strain. Use as a topical wash, as needed.

See also BARBERRY; BURDOCK; COMFREY; OCOTILLO BARK; OREGON GRAPE; SLIPPERY ELM; WHITE OAK; *and* YELLOW DOCK *in Part One.*

Ringworm

Ringworm (*Tinea corporis*) is a fungal infection but, despite its name, is not caused by worms. This skin infection is marked by pink-to-red circular lesions that have raised borders. The lesions tend to be clear in the center and expand outward. Medical doctors treat ringworm with topical antifungal preparations such as miconazole; however, certain herbs are also effective at eliminating this condition.

SECRETS
OF NATIVE
AMERICAN
HERBAL
REMEDIES

178

In addition to those herbs listed below, other beneficial herbs include sarsaparilla and yellow dock.

RINGWORM TEA #1

1 teaspoon echinacea root
1 teaspoon pau d'arco bark
2 cups boiling water

Combine the above herbs in a nonmetallic container and cover with the boiling water; steep for 30 minutes; strain. Take up to one cup per day.

TOPICAL WASH

1 teaspoon pau d'arco bark
1 teaspoon white cedar leaf tips
2 cups water

Place the above herbs in a glass container and cover with the water; let soak overnight; strain. Use topically, as needed.

See also ECHINACEA; PAU D'ARCO; SARSPARILLA; WHITE CEDAR LEAF TIPS; *and* YELLOW DOCK *in Part One.*

Scars

(*See* Wounds)

Sinusitis

Sinusitis is an inflammation of the sinuses, marked by sinus congestion, headache, and pain around the eyes or cheeks. There may be a nasal dis-

HEALING
INDIAN
FORMULAS
FOR INDIVIDUAL
CONDITIONS

179

charge, fatigue, cough, fever, earache, and an increased susceptibility to nasal infections.

Sinusitis can be caused by allergies, bacterial or fungal infections, and viral infections (such as the common cold). However, nasal injury, a deviated septum (the separator between the two nasal passages), a swollen conchae (the spiral air warmers in the nose), nasal polyps, or narrow sinuses can also cause sinusitis, as can cigarette smoke, dusty or dry air, or even infected tonsils or teeth.

In addition to those herbs listed below, other helpful herbs include elderberry, ginger, *Ginkgo biloba*, ginseng, licorice, marshmallow, pau d'arco, rose hips, slippery elm, valerian, wild indigo, and witch hazel.

SINUSITIS RELIEF TEA #1

1 teaspoon echinacea root
1 teaspoon yerba mansa root
1 teaspoon goldenseal root
1 cup boiling water

Combine the above herbs. Take two teaspoons of the mixture and cover with the boiling water; steep for 20 to 30 minutes; strain. Take warm, up to one cup per day, as needed.

SINUSITIS RELIEF TEA #2

1 teaspoon bayberry root
1 teaspoon white willow bark
2 cups boiling water

Combine the above herbs and cover with the boiling water; steep for 15 minutes; take warm, up to two cups a day.

See also BAYBERRY; BLACK ELDER; ECHINACEA; GINGER; *GINKGO BILOBA*; GINSENG; GOLDENSEAL; LICORICE; MARSHMALLOW; PAU D'ARCO; ROSE; SLIP-

SECRETS
OF NATIVE
AMERICAN
HERBAL
REMEDIES

180

PERY ELM; VALERIAN; WHITE WILLOW; WILD INDIGO ROOT; WITCH HAZEL; *and* YERBA MANSA *in Part One.*

Skin Rash

A skin rash is a temporary eruption on the skin that usually looks like small red or pink bumps. It may or may not itch. There may be scaly, round, or oval patches on the skin. A rash is usually a symptom of some other condition and can indicate a disease such as measles or chickenpox, an insect bite, an allergic reaction, a nutritional deficiency, or even dry skin.

In addition to those herbs listed below, other beneficial herbs include evening primrose, goldenseal, marshmallow, and strawberry.

SKIN RASH TEA

1 teaspoon burdock root
1 teaspoon Oregon grape root
1 teaspoon echinacea root
1 teaspoon yellow dock root
2 cups water

Combine the above herbs in a pan and cover with the water. Bring to a boil; reduce heat and simmer for 10 to 15 minutes; cool and strain. Take a tablespoon at a time, up to half a cup a day.

TOPICAL TEA

1 teaspoon comfrey root
1 teaspoon white oak leaves or bark
1 teaspoon slippery elm bark
2 cups water

Place the herbs in a container and cover with the water; bring to a boil and boil for 20 to 30 minutes; cool and strain. Use as a topical wash, as needed.

See also Burdock; Comfrey; Echinacea; Evening Primrose; Golden-seal; Marshmallow; Oregon Grape; Slippery Elm; Strawberry; White Oak; *and* Yellow Dock *in Part One; and* Allergies; Bites and Stings, Insect; Chickenpox; *and* Measles *in Part Two.*

Sore Throat

Usually, a sore throat is a minor problem that takes care of itself with time. Although we may not always be able to identify the cause of a sore throat, it most often occurs because of viral infections such as the flu or a common cold. It can also occur because of exposure to irritants such as dust or smoke, from allergies, or even from talking or yelling too loudly. A sore throat may make swallowing difficult and may lead to a hoarse voice.

In addition to those herbs listed below, other beneficial herbs to help relieve the pain of a sore throat include balsam fir, bayberry, blue vervain, cayenne, comfrey, coltsfoot, Indian root, marshmallow, osha root, Seneca snakeroot, and witch hazel.

SORE THROAT TEA

1 teaspoon Canadian fleabane leaves

1 teaspoon slippery elm bark

1 teaspoon echinacea root

2 cups boiling water

Combine the herbs in a nonmetallic container and cover with the boiling water; steep for 20 to 30 minutes; strain. Take up to two cups per day, warm.

SECRETS
OF NATIVE
AMERICAN
HERBAL
REMEDIES

182

SORE THROAT GARGLE

1 tablespoon elderberry fruit juice

1 tablespoon sumac extract

1 teaspoon echinacea root extract

Combine the above ingredients and gargle, as needed.

SORE THROAT LOZENGE

1 teaspoon goldenrod leaves

1 teaspoon wild cherry bark

1 teaspoon licorice root

1 teaspoon yerba sante leaves

1 teaspoon slippery elm bark

2 cups water

3 cups sugar

3 tablespoons corn syrup

Place the above herbs in a pan and cover with the water. Bring the mixture to a boil and boil for 20 minutes. Remove from the heat and cool. Strain the solution and add the sugar and the corn syrup. Place back on the heat, bring to a boil, then reduce heat to medium. Cook until the mixture reaches 300°F (hard-crack stage). Pour the syrup onto a large, buttered baking sheet; cool, then break into one-inch pieces. Use as you would any cough drop.

See also BALSAM FIR; BAYBERRY; BLACK ELDER; BLUE VERVAIN; CANADIAN FLEABANE; CAYENNE; COLTSFOOT; COMFREY; ECHINACEA; GOLDENROD; INDIAN ROOT; LICORICE; MARSHMALLOW; OSHA ROOT; SENECA SNAKEROOT; SLIPPERY ELM; SUMAC; WILD CHERRY; WITCH HAZEL; *and* YERBA SANTE *in Part One; and* ALLERGIES; COUGHS AND COLDS; INFLUENZA; LARYNGITIS; *and* TONSILLITIS *in Part Two.*

HEALING
INDIAN
FORMULAS
FOR INDIVIDUAL
CONDITIONS

183

Sprains and Strains

A sprain occurs when a ligament is severely wrenched, while a strain is a tearing and overstretching of muscle fibers. The same injuries that can cause a sprain can cause a strain as well. The difference is that a *sprain* involves ligaments and tendons, while a *strain* involves muscles. Sprains and strains are very common and can cause pain, swelling, bruising, and inflammation. Movement in the affected area is often limited because of the pain and/or swelling.

Most sprains and strains may heal without complications. But more severe injuries can become chronic, develop scar tissue, limit motion, and ultimately cause problems in surrounding tissues, nerves, vessels, and organs.

In addition to those herbs listed below, other helpful herbs include big sagebrush, bilberry, black currants, *Ginkgo biloba,* gotu kola, horsetail, licorice, marshmallow, and valerian.

TOPICAL PAIN RELIEF

20 drops yerba mansa tincture
4 ounces wintergreen oil
1 pound petroleum jelly

Thoroughly mix the above herbs with the petroleum jelly. Use as an ointment to relieve muscle pain.

PAIN RELIEF TEA #1

2 teaspoons black cohosh root
1 tablespoon ginseng root
2 cups water

Place the above herbs in a pan and cover with the water; bring to a boil; reduce heat and simmer for 30 minutes; cool and strain. Take two to three tablespoons, up to six times a day.

SECRETS
OF NATIVE
AMERICAN
HERBAL
REMEDIES

184

PAIN RELIEF TEA #2

1 tablespoon raspberry leaves

1 teaspoon white willow bark

2 cups boiling water

Combine the above herbs and cover with the boiling water; steep for 30 minutes; strain. Take as needed.

See also BIG SAGEBRUSH; BILBERRY; BLACK COHOSH; BLACK CURRANT; *GINKGO BILOBA*; GINSENG; GOTU KOLA; HORSETAIL; LICORICE; MARSHMAL-LOW; RASPBERRY; VALERIAN; WHITE WILLOW; WINTERGREEN; *and* YERBA MANSA *in Part One.*

Steatorrhea

Steatorrhea is the existence of excessive fat in the feces and is marked by soft, pale, malodorous, and bulky stools. Steatorrhea is actually more of a symptom than a disease and is a sign that your digestive system is not adequately breaking down the fat in your diet.

Steatorrhea can occur if you are deficient in certain enzymes (particularly the lipases), and it is a symptom of several conditions, including celiac disease, cystic fibrosis, pancreatic disease, and tropical sprue. When no cause can be determined, the condition is called "idiopathic steatorrhea" or nontropical sprue.

In addition to those herbs listed below, other beneficial herbs include chaparral and ocotillo bark.

STEATORRHEA TEA

1 teaspoon Oregon grape root

1 teaspoon yellow dock root

2 cups water

Combine the above herbs in a pan and cover with the water; bring to a boil and boil for several minutes; strain. Take up to one cup per day.

See also CHAPARRAL; OCOTILLO BARK; OREGON GRAPE; *and* YELLOW DOCK *in Part One.*

Stress

Increased heart rate, elevated blood pressure, muscle tension, irritability, depression, stomachache, and indigestion are all signs of stress. To many people, stress means emotional stress. But stress can also be physical (such as the injuries that occur because of a car accident or surgery) and biochemical (including exposure to pesticides or pollution and even poor nutrition). These (and other causes) make the body produce increased amounts of adrenaline. This is how the body copes with stress. But the adrenaline release also causes the heart rate to increase, blood pressure to rise, and muscles to tense.

A host of conditions can develop when the body is subjected to prolonged stress. These include an increased rate of aging, reduced resistance to infection, weakened immune function (which, in turn, can lead to other conditions such as chronic fatigue syndrome), and hormone overproduction (which can lead to adrenal fatigue).

A well-balanced diet and lifestyle can help anyone to better fight off the effects of stress.

NERVE TEA #1

1 teaspoon betony leaves

1 teaspoon kava kava root

1 teaspoon hops

1 teaspoon dried skullcap

1 cup boiling water

SECRETS
OF NATIVE
AMERICAN
HERBAL
REMEDIES

186

Combine the above herbs in a nonmetallic container. Put two teaspoons of the mixture in another such container and cover with the boiling water; steep for 30 minutes; cool and strain. Take one tablespoon at a time, as needed.

NERVE TEA #2

1 teaspoon powdered ginger
1 teaspoon powdered valerian root
1 teaspoon powdered pleurisy root
2 cups boiling water

Combine the above herbs in a nonmetallic container and cover with the boiling water; steep for 30 minutes; cool and strain. Take one tablespoon at a time, as needed, up to two cups a day.

NERVE TEA #3

1 to 2 teaspoons peppermint leaves
1 teaspoon valerian root
1 cup boiling water

Combine the above ingredients and cover with the boiling water; steep for 20 to 30 minutes; strain. Drink up to one cup per day, as needed.

See also BETONY; GINGER; HOPS; KAVA KAVA; PEPPERMINT; PLEURISY ROOT; SKULL CAP; *and* VALERIAN *in Part One.*

Sunburn

A sunburn can occur when we stay out in the sun too long. The red skin that is characteristic of a sunburn usually occurs between one and twenty-four hours

HEALING
INDIAN
FORMULAS
FOR INDIVIDUAL
CONDITIONS

187

after exposure. Sunburns are marked by pain, swelling, and sometimes blisters. Fever, chills, weakness, and even shock may occur because of a severe sunburn.

Most experts advise using sunscreen to protect the skin from the sun's harmful rays. Sunscreens are rated by their sun protection factor (SPF). A sunscreen with an SPF of 30 gives twice the protection of one rated SPF 15.

Anyone with a severe sunburn should seek medical attention. Herbs can help relieve the pain of those with less severe sunburns.

SUNBURN RELIEF TEA

1 tablespoon chamomile flowers
1 teaspoon St. John's wort leaves
1 teaspoon echinacea root
2 cups boiling water

Combine the above herbs in a nonmetallic container and cover with the boiling water; steep for 30 minutes; cool and strain. Drink up to two cups a day.

TOPICAL SUNBURN RELIEF

1 teaspoon coneflower root
1 teaspoon goldenrod leaves
1 teaspoon echinacea root
1 cup boiling water

Combine the above herbs in a nonmetallic container and cover with the boiling water. Steep for 30 minutes; cool and strain. Apply as a wash, as needed.

See also CHAMOMILE; CONEFLOWER; ECHINACEA; GOLDENROD; *and* ST. JOHN'S WORT *in Part One.*

SECRETS
OF NATIVE
AMERICAN
HERBAL
REMEDIES

188

Thrush

Thrush is a fungal infection of the mouth caused by *Candida albicans*, the same fungus that causes candidiasis. Thrush looks like creamy white patches that appear on the lining of the mouth and on the tongue. The patches can be scraped off. The usual treatment for thrush is topical application of a drug called nystatin, but herbs are often just as effective. In addition to those herbs listed below, another beneficial herb is osha root.

Children with thrush should be under the care of a qualified health-care practitioner.

THRUSH TEA

2 teaspoons big sagebrush root
1 tablespoon pau d'arco bark
1 cup water

Place the above herbs in a glass container and cover with the water; let soak overnight; strain. Take a mouthful at a time, swishing the liquid in your mouth for several minutes before swallowing.

See also BIG SAGEBRUSH; OSHA ROOT; *and* PAU D'ARCO *in Part One.*

Tonsillitis

Tonsillitis is an inflammation of the tonsils, usually caused by a viral or bacterial infection. Tonsillitis is marked by a painful sore throat and inflammation and redness in the back of the throat. The pain may make swallowing difficult. Additional symptoms include coughing, earache, fever, headache, hoarseness, nausea, and vomiting. Lymph nodes throughout the body may be enlarged. Tonsillitis is most frequently found in children, but it is possible to have tonsillitis at any age. Children with tonsillitis should be under the care of a qualified health-care practitioner.

HEALING
INDIAN
FORMULAS
FOR INDIVIDUAL
CONDITIONS

189

Tonics

Back in the days before refrigerators and freezers, most Native Americans survived winter by eating dried meats, fruits, and vegetables, and whatever they were able to hunt or fish. No wonder they looked forward to the advent of spring with its vitamin- and mineral-rich greens and the tonic their herbal healers made from fresh herbs. Most spring tonics not only served as diuretics but also provided much-needed nutrients.

In addition to those herbs listed below, other beneficial herbs to use in tonics include chicory, dandelion, ginseng, goldenseal, ground ivy, lady's slipper, passionflower, peppermint, raspberry, red willow, sarsaparilla, Solomon's seal, wild cherry, yarrow, yellow dock, and yucca.

TONIC #1

1 teaspoon black cohosh root

1 teaspoon stone root

1 teaspoon elecampane root

3 cups water

Honey

Combine the above herbs in a pan and cover with the water. Bring to a boil and boil for 30 minutes; cool and strain. You may want to sweeten with honey. Take two to three tablespoons, up to six times a day.

TONIC #2

2 tablespoons Oregon grape root

2 tablespoons wild cherry bark

2 cups water

Place the above herbs in a pan; cover with the water. Bring to a boil; boil for 20 to 30 minutes; cool and strain. Take twice a day, a tablespoon or two at a time.

SECRETS
OF NATIVE
AMERICAN
HERBAL
REMEDIES

190

In addition to those herbs listed below, other beneficial herbs to help relieve the pain of tonsillitis and strengthen the body to better fight infection include balsam fir, bayberry, blue vervain, cayenne, coltsfoot, comfrey, goldenseal, Indian root, marshmallow, osha root, sage, Seneca snakeroot, valerian, white willow bark, wild indigo root, and witch hazel.

TONSILLITIS TEA

1 teaspoon Canadian fleabane leaves
1 teaspoon slippery elm bark
1 teaspoon echinacea root
2 cups boiling water

Combine the above herbs and cover with the boiling water; steep for 20 to 30 minutes; strain. Take up to two cups per day, warm.

TONSILLITIS GARGLE

1 tablespoon elderberry fruit juice
1 tablespoon sumac extract
1 teaspoon echinacea root extract

Combine the above ingredients and gargle, as needed.

TONSILLITIS LOZENGES

1 teaspoon goldenrod leaves
1 teaspoon wild cherry bark
1 teaspoon licorice root
1 teaspoon yerba sante leaves
1 teaspoon slippery elm bark
2 cups water
3 cups sugar
3 tablespoons corn syrup

HEALING
INDIAN
FORMULAS
FOR INDIVIDUAL
CONDITIONS

191

Place the above herbs in a pan and cover with the water. Bring the mixture to a boil and boil for 20 minutes. Remove from the heat and cool. Strain the solution and add the sugar and the corn syrup. Place back on the heat, bring to a boil, then reduce heat to medium. Cook until the mixture reaches 300°F (hard-crack stage). Pour the syrup onto a large, buttered baking sheet; cool, then break into one-inch pieces. Use as you would any cough drop.

See also Balsam Fir; Bayberry; Black Elder; Blue Vervain; Canadian Fleabane; Cayenne; Coltsfoot; Comfrey; Echinacea; Goldenrod; Goldenseal; Indian Root; Licorice; Marshmallow; Osha Root; Sage; Seneca Snakeroot; Slippery Elm; Sumac; Valerian; White Willow; Wild Cherry; Wild Indigo; Witch Hazel; *and* Yerba Sante *in Part One; and* Coughs and Colds; Ear Infections; Fever; Laryngitis; *and* Sore Throat *in Part Two.*

Toothache

Toothache can be caused by any number of problems, including decaying teeth, sensitivity to heat or cold, or excessive pressure on the tooth. Sometimes tooth pain occurs because of sinusitis, when pressure from the inflamed sinuses presses on nerves that run to the teeth.

It is especially important to seek dental care if a toothache occurs because of tooth decay. This is because tooth decay can spread infection throughout the body.

PAIN RELIEF TEA

1 tablespoon raspberry leaves
1 teaspoon white willow bark
2 cups boiling water

Combine the above herbs and cover with the boiling water; steep for 30 minutes; strain. Take as needed, up to one cup a day.

CAVITY PREVENTION WASH

1 teaspoon bayberry root bark
1 teaspoon goldenseal root
1 teaspoon chaparral leaves
2 cups water

Combine the above ingredients in a pan and cover with the water; bring to a boil and boil for 15 minutes; cool and strain. To use, place one to two tablespoons of the solution in your mouth and swish around. Hold in your mouth as long as possible before spitting out. Use as needed.

See also BAYBERRY; CHAPARRAL; GOLDENSEAL; RASPBERRY; *and* WHITE WILLOW *in Part One; and* SINUSITIS *in Part Two.*

Tuberculosis (TB)

Tuberculosis (formerly called "consumption") is a chronic, recurrent infection that most often affects the lungs, although any organ may be affected. Tuberculosis is caused by bacteria such as *Mycobacterium tuberculosis, M. africanum,* or *M. bovis.* After the invention of antibiotics, tuberculosis was almost eliminated. Unfortunately, however, because of the AIDS epidemic, TB incidence is on the increase. In fact, some authorities believe we are close to a potentially dangerous tuberculosis epidemic. In addition, the bacteria that cause TB are now becoming resistant to the antibiotics usually used to treat them.

Before antibiotics, people used herbs to treat tuberculosis. In addition to those herbs listed below, other herbs that can help relieve some of the symptoms of TB include barberry, coltsfoot, horsetail, and goldenrod.

HEALING
INDIAN
FORMULAS
FOR INDIVIDUAL
CONDITIONS

193

TUBERCULOSIS SYRUP

1 teaspoon elecampane root
1 teaspoon sage leaves
1 teaspoon goldenseal root
1 teaspoon Solomon's seal
1 teaspoon horehound leaves
3 cups water
1 pound honey

Combine the above herbs in a pan and cover with the water; bring to a boil and boil for 20 minutes; strain. Combine the tea with the honey and heat on low. Stir to dissolve the honey; when dissolved, remove the mixture from the heat. When cool, pour into glass containers and seal. Take two tablespoons at a time, as needed.

See also BARBERRY; COLTSFOOT; ELECAMPANE; GOLDENROD; GOLDENSEAL; HOREHOUND; HORSETAIL; SAGE; *and* SOLOMON'S SEAL *in Part One.*

Ulcers, Skin

(*See* Bed Sores)

Uterine Fibroids

(*See* Dysmenorrhea)

Varicose Veins

Varicose veins are abnormally enlarged veins that appear close to the skin's surface. They occur primarily in the calves and thighs and result from

SECRETS
OF NATIVE
AMERICAN
HERBAL
REMEDIES

194

obstruction of the veins or from prolonged pressure. Varicose veins can develop from long periods of standing or sitting, as well as lack of exercise, pregnancy, excessive weight, and prolonged constipation, and from conditions such as phlebitis. Heredity is also a factor for many individuals.

Varicose veins are very common and affect approximately 10 percent of the population. They can be painful and often cause cramping of the leg muscles and ankle swelling.

CIRCULATORY TEA

2 teaspoons black cohosh root

4 teaspoons Ginkgo biloba *leaves*

2 cups boiling water

Combine the above herbs. Pour the boiling water over the herb mixture; soak for 30 minutes; strain. Take two to three tablespoons at a time, up to six times a day, to improve circulation.

TOPICAL WASH

1 teaspoon ocotillo bark

1 teaspoon yarrow

1 teaspoon witch hazel bark

2 cups water

Combine the above herbs in a pan and cover with the water; bring to a boil and boil until reduced to one cup; cool and strain. To relieve discomfort, apply topically, as needed.

See also BLACK COHOSH; *GINKGO BILOBA*; OCOTILLO BARK; WITCH HAZEL; *and* YARROW *in Part One; and* CIRCULATORY DISORDERS; CONSTIPATION; *and* OBESITY *in Part Two.*

HEALING
INDIAN
FORMULAS
FOR INDIVIDUAL
CONDITIONS

195

Vomiting

(*See* Nausea and Vomiting)

Wounds

Most wounds are caused by cuts, abrasions, or other physical injuries. Wounds should always to cleaned thoroughly to avoid an infection. The bleeding that often accompanies a wound can usually be stopped by applying pressure to the wound. Excessive bleeding, or injury to major arteries, requires immediate emergency medical care. If a wound turns red, swells, throbs, or is hot to the touch and contains pus, it is a sign of infection. In addition to those herbs listed below, other beneficial herbs to treat wounds include black currants, blue vervain, chamomile, echinacea, feverfew, goldenrod, goldenseal, horsetail, marshmallow, mullein, oxeye daisy, St. John's wort, slippery elm, speedwell, witch hazel, and yarrow.

WOUND TOPICAL APPLICATION

1 teaspoon white pine inner bark

1 teaspoon wild cherry bark

1 teaspoon wild plum root

2 cups water

Combine the above herbs in a pan and cover with the water. Bring to a boil and boil until the bark and roots are soft. Cool and strain. To use, soak a clean cloth in the solution and apply to the affected area.

FOR CUTS

1 teaspoon pleurisy root

1 teaspoon ginseng root

2 cups water

SECRETS
OF NATIVE
AMERICAN
HERBAL
REMEDIES

196

Combine the above herbs in a pan and cover with the water; bring to a boil and boil for 20 to 30 minutes; strain. Apply topically, as needed.

See also BLACK CURRANT; BLUE VERVAIN; CHAMOMILE; ECHINACEA; FEVER-FEW; GINSENG; GOLDENROD; GOLDENSEAL; HORSETAIL; MARSHMALLOW; MULLEIN; OXEYE DAISY; PINE; PLEURISY ROOT; ST. JOHN'S WORT; SLIPPERY ELM; SPEEDWELL; WILD CHERRY; WILD PLUM; WITCH HAZEL; *and* YARROW *in Part One.*

Yeast Infections

(*See* Candidiasis)

HEALING
INDIAN
FORMULAS
FOR INDIVIDUAL
CONDITIONS

197

PART THREE

Healing Medicine and the Power of the Great Spirit

Although this book is about herbal healing, herbs are only one part of the overall Native American philosophy of health. At the heart of Native American healing is a trust and belief in a higher power—the Great Spirit, the Creator— and the role He plays in our everyday lives. Each tribe or nation has its own name for this Great Spirit. The Arapaho call It "Man Above," the Pawnees refer to It as "Ti-rá-wa," the Crows speak of It as "First Maker," and the Sioux call It "The Great Spirit" or "Mystery."

The animals, the plants, water . . . everything in nature are gifts entrusted to us by our Creator. According to American Indians, if properly cared for, these gifts will feed us, clothe and shelter us, care for us when we are sick or injured, and keep us healthy. But these gifts bring responsibilities to care for and to respect nature and the universe and to use these gifts only as needed. People are an essential part of the universe, but only a part of a whole, lovingly fashioned by the Creator. Almost every Native American culture believes that everything—every animal, living creature, plant, rock, tree, mountain, and even water—has a soul. Therefore, all of nature must be treated with respect and honored.

E. Thomas Morning Owl, language program coordinator of the Confederated Tribes of the Umatilla [Oregon] Indian Reservation, says that when raised around Native American elders, one not only learns the language and the religious practices of their respective tribe but also how to look at plants, animals, and even inanimate objects holistically. One learns that everything has a soul and that even a rock has a spirit and a purpose. "When I was young," Morning Owl relates, "I was walking along a creek with my grandmother. I bent over, grabbed a rock, and threw it into the water. Immediately my grandmother asked me, 'Why did you do that? How long did it take that rock to get out of the water? And you put it right back in there? Why did you put it back in the water? It wasn't bothering you. You had no reason to do that, do you realize that?' " This and other lessons helped shape Morning Owl's view of the world around him and his relationship with nature.

According to Morning Owl, because Indians respect nature and the environment, many people think that Native Americans think they have all the answers. "We do not," he says. "But our people have had to live within nature, so we're very in tune to it. Fortunately, many Native American people are still in tune with nature. They still know how to listen and what to watch for in the changing cycles of nature. Some people still teach the way my elders, my mother, my grandmother, and all the people in my life did—those people who helped fashion my way of life when I was growing up. Those people taught me that we are not separate from nature, but part of it. It is part of our religious point of view.

"To Native Americans, we don't have dominion over anything. These creatures in nature were all here prior to when humans were placed on this earth. Therefore, we are not above any plants or animals, but it is the plants and animals that take care of people. Native Americans recognize that everything has an ordained spirit and that humans are not at the center of nature, but an essential part of the whole."

SECRETS
OF NATIVE
AMERICAN
HERBAL
REMEDIES

200

There is, therefore, a balance in life, an essential balance between the plants, animals, rocks, water, and everything else—even of and within humans. With every breath of life, Native Americans strive to be in harmony with nature and the universe by harnessing the energy around them to improve and prolong life. "All things in balance" is not only the American Indian philosophy of life, it is their *way* of life.

But sometimes this balance is disturbed. Loss of balance within the body weakens the body and can result in illness. Therefore, the first step in returning to wellness is to discover why you're out of balance; only then can you restore balance.

James Bowman, D.C., D.Ht., is part Lakota Sioux, part Navajo, and of Western European heritage. A highly respected chiropractor practicing in Stevens Point, Wisconsin (his Navajo name as a healer is Medicine Hand, while his Lakota name is Talks Like Grass), Dr. Bowman is a director of the American Preventive Medical Association and an authority on alternative health care. His upbringing, combined with his professional training, has given him powerful insights into Native American health and healing. According to Dr. Bowman, although disease might result from injury or infection, this overt event is not the true, original cause of the illness. The cause is loss of balance. "Balance is always the key in everything," he says. "Injury and illness are not seen as disjointed or disconnected events, but as aspects of the whole life experience."

Native Americans believe that certain underlying causes can make an individual more vulnerable to disease or injury. According to Dr. Bowman, "When you have left the land, your people, your ways, your life; and when in thought, word, or deed you have given away your power, your identity, your reverence, and especially your humility before Almighty God, the Great Spirit, the Creator of the entire living universe; when you are careless with the gifts with which you have been entrusted; when you are irresponsible in your duties; when you place your own small individual self above the Creator, or above your tribal members, above their good, then you are vulnerable. [Once you leave] the path of sacred reverence [of] creation you lose perspective, humil-

HEALING
MEDICINE
AND THE
POWER OF THE
GREAT SPIRIT

201

ity, understanding, and power; you lose the good things and you become vulnerable. Lying, stealing, dishonest interpersonal dealings, not being a person of your word, putting on airs (that is, being someone or something you are not), being arrogant, [makes you] vulnerable. In essence, whenever you damage or break the sacredness of life, you violate the sacred principle and you suffer. If you cause another to suffer through your negligence or carelessness, much less through your intentional wish to harm them, you suffer and you become responsible for rectifying your own suffering, as well as the suffering which you cause to others.

"Suffering comes perhaps in the form of guilt, shame, anger, damaged relationships, insomnia, ulcers, headaches, etc.," says Dr. Bowman. "Suffering occurs until the causes are identified and resolution through rebalancing is achieved. Much of this has to do with getting one's spirit, that is, one's heart, mind, emotions, and attitude, 'right'; by asking for forgiveness; by showing and accepting forgiveness; by making a sincere commitment to right the wrong, leave the destructive ways, and rejoin the balanced life; by being a person of integrity and responsibility; and by doing the right thing. But you can only do the right thing when you are balanced in your heart, mind, and spirit. Negative thinking and feelings can cause a darkness in the heart or mind, clouding judgment and undermining your return to balance. So, in effect, suffering is also a gift from nature because suffering causes one to think, repent, make necessary changes, and become balanced again."

Native Americans certainly believe that their emotions can have an effect on their health, and modern science is beginning to agree. We now know that emotional stress can affect your body's physical health. Emotional stress causes the adrenal glands to release hormones, increasing blood flow to the muscles, while simultaneously restricting blood flow to the kidneys and the stomach. Nerve and hormonal activity increases and muscles tense. This is all part of the "fight-or-flight" reaction. Unfortunately, modern Americans don't fight or run away from confrontation; instead our muscles store up this tension, which prevents them from relaxing. They then develop spasms and pain.

SECRETS
OF NATIVE
AMERICAN
HERBAL
REMEDIES

202

We also get heartburn because we're upset, and our blood pressure rises. In short, our emotions have altered our health.

What can you learn from the Native Americans to help heal your body, your mind, and your spirit? We can learn that healing the body must first begin with healing the spirit. Although physical cures, such as the use of herbs, can help, spiritual healing is much more important to the American Indian and must come first. True healing can only occur when the body and spirit are in balance. Herbs are more effective when the mind and spirit are balanced and healthy.

Native Americans have used a variety of means to heal the spirit. However, using any of these methods, the goal is to enlist the Creator's help, because only through the Great Spirit is healing possible. The medicine man, of course, is the channel through which God works. It is the medicine man's responsibility to drive off disease-causing bad influences and evil spirits. Spirit uses him as a vessel to heal the sick. To be more receptive to God's message, the medicine man might set himself apart for days at a time, cleansing himself through meditation, prayer, and fasting. The medicine man uses chants, dances, prayers, sweats, sand paintings, and other means to help return balance and heal the sick or injured. He might even apply his mouth directly to the area of illness and suck out the evil that caused the pain and spit "it" onto the ground.

Sometimes medicine women or herbal healers might also be involved. Although the women of the tribes generally seem to be most familiar with the herbal brews and potions, the knowledge of herbal medicine is certainly not confined to women. Women often learn how to use herbs from their mothers and grandmothers, or from their husbands, if they happen to be medicine men.

Regardless of who helps to channel God's healing energy, Native American healing is very individualistic. What works for one individual might not work for somebody else, even if they have the same condition, because the causes can vary, as can the individual's spirit, nature, and personality. In addition, those living in different geographic areas have access to different herbs and healing practices than those living in other areas. For instance, the plants that grow in the desert are not the same plants that grow on the plains, in the mountains, along the rivers, or on the seashore. But regardless of what herbs or other practices are used, the goal is always to address the whole person—body, mind, and spirit.

Although they had no research centers and no huge government grants, over the centuries, Native Americans have developed, often through trial and error, a proven method of healing, unrivaled by present-day "scientific" medicine. There is evidence that American Indians long ago developed syringes and enema bags; they also knew about anesthetics and how to set broken bones. Their method of healing combines faith, prayer, and the use of gifts provided by the Creator, including plants, animals, and water.

You probably don't have a medicine man down the street to help you return balance to your body, mind, and spirit. So how can you integrate Native American healing practices into your own therapy program? Years ago, I developed the Five-Step Jump-Start Program that utilizes all of the aspects of Native American healing to help people take charge of their lives and their health.

The Five-Step Jump-Start Program encompasses five key areas: detoxification, proper diet, nutritional supplements including herbs, exercise, and a positive mental attitude. However, it is essential to understand that each step must deal with the body, the mind, and the spirit simultaneously, in order to succeed. Therefore, some form of prayer and spirituality should always be involved.

For more information on the spiritual aspect of healing, see the following books:

American Indian Medicine by Virgil J. Vogel (Norman: University of Oklahoma Press, 1970).

Earthway by Mary Summer Rain (New York: Pocket Books, 1990).

The Medicine Men, Oglala Sioux Ceremony and Healing by Thomas H. Lewis (Lincoln: University of Nebraska Press, 1990).

Secrets of the Sacred White Buffalo by Gary Null (Paramus, NJ: Prentice Hall, 1998).

SECRETS
OF NATIVE
AMERICAN
HERBAL
REMEDIES

204

Shamanic Healing and Ritual Drama by Åake Hultkrantz (New York: Crossroad, 1992).

Spirit Healing by Mary Dean Atwood (New York: Sterling, 1991).

Detoxification

Detoxification is the first step of the plan. For centuries, Native Americans have used sweat lodges and fasting as ways to benefit from the healing properties of detoxification. Of all the purification ceremonies in North America, the sweat lodge ceremony is the most widespread. The Lakota call the ceremony *inikagapi*, and the Chippewa called the sweat bath ritual a *madodoson*. The Apache called the sweat lodge itself *taachi*, while the Cheyenne called it *vonhäom*. Similar in action to a sauna, the sweat lodge's heat and moisture help detoxify the body—mentally, physically, and spiritually. The smoke in the lodge and the ceremonial rituals conducted there all contribute to the native healing process.

Sweat lodges have at least nine health-giving functions:

1. In the sweat lodge, healing can begin for many physical or emotional disorders. It is an opportunity to pray, speak, and ask for forgiveness from the Creator, as well as from other people who have been previously hurt.

2. The cleansing heat increases body temperature, thereby increasing the body's enzymatic activity. This increased activity helps the body destroy viruses and bacteria and stimulates immune function. The famous Greek physician Hippocrates once said, "Give me a fever and I can cure any disease." Increased temperatures help the body to practically burn away bacterial and viral agents and illnesses.

3. Physically, sweating helps detoxify the body by opening any clogged pores and allowing elimination of internal toxins, heavy metals, excessive urea, and metabolic by-products.

4. As the body's temperature rises, endocrine glandular function is stimulated. This helps to cleanse the body and improve body function.

5. The heat of the sweat lodge dilates the large blood vessels and capillaries which, in turn, stimulates increased blood flow to the skin and increases the rate at which the body's organs are flushed of toxins.

6. The moist air of the sweat lodge improves lung function. Clogged respiratory passages are dilated, giving relief from minor respiratory problems and colds. Caution: Individuals with major respiratory problems and pneumonia should not use the sweat lodge.

7. Hot water and steam created by pouring water over the rocks result in negative ion release. Positive ions are associated with tension and fatigue, as well as allergies, rheumatism, arthritis, insomnia, and asthma.

8. Sweat lodges can improve metabolic function. By removing toxins and other waste products, as well as improving circulation, the digestion, absorption, and utilization of herbs and other nutrients can be improved.

9. The sweat lodge can be a cleansing and regenerative experience, much like a rebirth. In his book *Sweat*, Mikkel Aaland observes, "The warm, dark, moist ambiance inside a sweat bath is easily likened to a womb, even the womb of Mother Earth, Herself."

Sweat lodges can be many different sizes and shapes and are constructed using materials found in the local environment. For example, tribes of the Southwest built circular subterranean sweat lodges in which individuals descended a ladder to the underground structure, which was encased in bedrock. Other tribes used mud, wood, or animal skins to build sweat lodges. Cedar planks were used in the far Northwest; buffalo skins covered the Plains Indians' sweat lodges, while skins or birch bark might cover frames made from willow poles in the Northeast. In the Southeast, sweat lodges might be dug into a hillside or built up into earth mounds. The polar Inuit Indians even used igloos as sweat lodges.

The sweat lodge typically holds ten to fifteen people comfortably and is

SECRETS
OF NATIVE
AMERICAN
HERBAL
REMEDIES

206

light-tight to ensure that they are in total darkness. Usually, hot rocks are heated on a fire and then brought into the sweat lodge. The ceremony leader then pours water onto the rocks to produce steam to encourage sweating and cleansing and to stimulate spiritual healing. Prayers are then recited, songs are sung, and the spirits are called into the lodge in an effort to purify the participants. The door is rarely opened during a ceremony, because the heat and dark are important to help the participants focus on what they are doing.

If a sweat lodge is not available, a sauna, such as those found at any health club, makes a good substitute. Or you can build your own sweat lodge. Follow the American Indian's example and use materials available in your own environment.

Do-It-Yourself Construction

1. First find the proper location to build your sweat lodge. The sweat lodge should be located close to a cool clear stream, lake, or river, or the ocean, since there must be a location to cool the body after being in the sweat lodge or sauna. If this is not possible, you can use your shower or bath to cool down after the sweat lodge.

2. Dig the pit. The pit should be in the very center of the structure and should be about two feet deep and two to three feet wide. This hole is extremely symbolic and even holy. To the Plains Indians, it traditionally represents the center of the universe.

3. Gather poles to use for the framework. Willows and other saplings work well for this purpose. Although there is no set size for a sweat lodge, gather sufficient poles to construct a lodge two to four feet high in the center and about ten feet in diameter.

4. To make the framework, plant the ends of the poles into the ground, joining the ends in the center (much like a dome in appearance). Use leather

HEALING
MEDICINE
AND THE
POWER OF THE
GREAT SPIRIT

207

string or rope to tie the ends together. Be sure to point the entrance of the lodge to the east toward Father Sun, who has tremendous power.

5. The next step is to cover the poles with material that will keep the heat in and the light out. Rather than the animal skins that used to be used to cover sweat lodges, you may need to use heavy duty canvas sheets.

6. To use the sweat lodge, you'll need to heat rocks. The best way to do this is in an outside pit. To the Creeks, the fire used to heat the rocks represents a portion of the sun and a symbol of the Creator. The stones used in the pit represent earth as both mother and grandmother and symbolize endurance, just as the earth endures.

7. Once the rocks have been brought into the sweat lodge and placed in the pit, water should be poured onto the rocks to produce steam. The water used in the sweat lodge represents the life-giving elements of air and water.

8. An offering should be made to the fire. Native Americans often used tobacco for this purpose.

9. Drinking herbal teas in the sweat lodge can help encourage healthy skin and sweating. Herbs used for this purpose include cayenne, elderberries, ginger, pepper, peppermint, sage, and wintergreen. Drink as much tea as possible while you sweat. This will also help replenish fluids the body loses during sweating.

10. Stay in the sweat lodge for about fifteen minutes.

After the sweat, wrap up in a blanket and cool in bed for thirty to sixty minutes. Then, plunge into a nearby stream, river, or other body of water. If this isn't possible, take a cold shower or bath instead.

SECRETS
OF NATIVE
AMERICAN
HERBAL
REMEDIES

208

Diet

Diet is the second part of the plan and involves eating fresh, enzyme-rich fruits and vegetables. This is another practice American Indians have followed for centuries. Although they had no word for enzymes, they were well aware that foods must be vital and alive in order that one remains healthy and full of energy. They picked foods in season; they knew there was a vital force that was in each object, be it plant, animal, or human. They knew this vital force was essential for life and that it came from the Creator to make life possible. We now know that the vital and alive force within foods is enzymes. Our body uses enzymes for every single chemical reaction. No plant, animal, vitamin, mineral, or hormone could do its work without enzymes. All the cells, tissues, and organs in our body are run by enzymes. Enzymes help build proteins and are essential for digestion, blood coagulation, and breathing, as well as every other bodily activity. Since enzymes trigger the conversion of nutritional substances into energy in every cell of the body, a proper intake of raw, enzyme-rich foods is essential. Like the traditional American Indian, eating fresh foods from animals or plant sources, harvested in season, ensures a healthier, more balanced body. For further information on enzymes and why they are so important to good health, see my book *The Complete Book of Enzyme Therapy* (Garden City Park, NY: Avery, 1999).

Fresh foods are extremely healthy foods for the body, yet respectful of nature. "Balance" is the key to proper health. In order to attain this balance chemically, foods must be eaten fresh and in season and only when you're hungry.

Fresh fruits and vegetables contain more enzymes, minerals, and vitamins than canned, frozen, or processed foods. This is because heat, chemicals, and long storage times can destroy or deplete the nutrients in these foods. Be in tune with nature: eat only foods that are grown organically and have not been genetically modified. Avoid food grown with artificial fertilizers, growth-stimulating chemicals, herbicides, or insecticides. If you find it hard to eat raw foods, use a wok to stir-fry them or steam or blanch them slightly. Avoid most restaurant foods, such as fried, frozen, and processed foods, as well as foods loaded with animal or other saturated fats, salt, preservatives, and sulfites. To aid digestion (as well as detoxification), drink fresh water with your meals.

Also avoid aluminum cookware and cooking utensils. Aluminum salts are

HEALING
MEDICINE
AND THE
POWER OF THE
GREAT SPIRIT

209

easily assimilated into the body because they are water-soluble. Use only stainless steel, iron, or glass cookware. Avoid coated cookware, as the materials used to coat the cookware may leach into the food.

Supplements Including Herbs

The third part of the plan, nutritional supplements, includes the use of herbs. Herbs are the subject of Part One of this book. See that section for detailed information on herbs and how they can improve your health.

Also important is a proper balance of vitamins, minerals, and enzymes; in fact, they are essential for life.

VITAMINS

Vitamins are organic food substances that are required for a wide variety of activities in your body, including antibody formation, blood coagulation, bone and tooth formation, growth, reproduction, resistance to infection, and formation and maintenance of healthy skin, bones, muscles, and nerves. In addition, many of your body's enzymes cannot function without vitamin "helpers." Vitamins are either fat-soluble or water-soluble. The B vitamins and vitamin C are water-soluble vitamins, absorbed from the intestine and excreted in urine, and must be replenished daily. Vitamins A, D, E, and K are fat-soluble vitamins. These vitamins are absorbed, transported, and metabolized along with fat. Unlike water-soluble vitamins, fat-soluble vitamins are not excreted (to any great extent) in urine. Instead, they are either eliminated in the feces or are absorbed and stored in fat and liver tissue. Since excretion of these vitamins is minimal, caution should be exercised when taking fat-soluble vitamin supplements, as toxicity can result. Follow the directions on the label for dosage information.

Vitamin A

♠ Vitamin A is a fat-soluble vitamin.

SECRETS
OF NATIVE
AMERICAN
HERBAL
REMEDIES

210

♠ Vitamin A is essential for proper vision, healthy skin, a strong immune system, and proper hair, bone, tooth, and nail development.

♠ Signs of a vitamin A deficiency include night blindness and dry, itching, and burning eyes. Other symptoms include dry skin and hair, defective taste and smell, appetite loss, exhaustion, and an increased susceptibility to infections (including respiratory, urogenital, and digestive infections).

♠ Food sources for vitamin A include dairy products (including milk, cheese, and butter), egg yolks, liver, and fish (such as herring, sardines, and tuna). Your body can convert the carotenoids in vegetables (such as broccoli, carrots, sweet potatoes, squash, and tomatoes) and fruits (such as cantaloupe, apricots, and peaches) into vitamin A.

Vitamin B_1 (thiamin)

♠ Vitamin B_1 is a water-soluble vitamin.

♠ Vitamin B_1 is essential for carbohydrate metabolism, proper energy production in the brain, nerve function, appetite, and heart function. Vitamin B_1 also supports muscles, hair, eyes, and hearing.

♠ Signs of a deficiency include weakness, fatigue, visual disturbances, edema, decreased appetite and other digestive disturbances, poor memory, confusion, sleep disturbances, constipation, muscle weakness, difficulty walking, calf muscle pain, lack of ankle or knee jerk reflexes, wrist drop and foot drop, numbness of the hands and feet, heart problems (such as abnormal rhythms, enlarged heart, or even heart failure), paralysis, irritability, nervousness, mental depression, and shortness of breath.

♠ Food sources include carbohydrate-rich foods (such as legumes, whole grains, enriched breads and cereals, seeds, nuts, and the germ of cereal grains), brewer's yeast, and meats (such as pork, ham, bacon, and liver).

Vitamin B$_2$ (riboflavin)

♠ Vitamin B$_2$ is a water-soluble vitamin.

♠ Vitamin B$_2$ supports vision, mucous membrane integrity, and healthy skin, nails, and hair.

♠ Signs of a deficiency include gastrointestinal tract problems; dermatitis (skin rash); anemia; cracking at the corners of the mouth; inflamed, purple-red, shiny tongue; visual problems (such as light sensitivity, burning eyes, blurred vision, inflamed eyelids, corneal reddening, and cataract formation); poor digestion; premature wrinkles; and retarded growth. Oral contraceptives may increase the need for riboflavin.

♠ Food sources include meat (especially organ meats, such as liver, heart, and kidney), milk, yogurt, cottage cheese, eggs, whole grains, and leafy, green vegetables.

Vitamin B$_3$ (niacin)

♠ Vitamin B$_3$ is a water-soluble vitamin.

♠ Vitamin B$_3$ is important in energy metabolism. It also stimulates gastric juices and hydrochloric acid, maintains the nervous system and brain, and supports healthy skin, liver, and gastrointestinal tract. "Niacin" is the collective term used in referring to nicotinic acid and its amide, nicotinamide.

♠ Signs of a deficiency include headache, loss of appetite, listlessness, and pellagra (characterized by dermatitis, mucous membrane inflammation, gastrointestinal problems, canker sores, and mental disturbances, including depression, confusion, delusions, disorientation, and hallucinations).

♠ Niacin-rich foods are widely distributed in animal and plant foods, including meats, organ meats (such as liver), fish, and poultry, milk, vegetables (such as legumes and green leafy vegetables), whole grains (except corn), brewer's yeast, and even tea and coffee.

SECRETS
OF NATIVE
AMERICAN
HERBAL
REMEDIES

212

Vitamin B$_5$ (pantothenic acid)

♠ Vitamin B$_5$ is a water-soluble vitamin.

♠ Pantothenic acid (from the Greek word meaning "universal") is converted in the body to coenzyme A, important in the metabolism of protein, fats, and carbohydrates. It is also involved in the synthesis of hormones, hemoglobin, steroids, and neurotransmitters (such as acetylcholine) and is needed for the digestive system, skin, adrenal glands, and the brain.

♠ Signs of a deficiency include fatigue, insomnia, loss of appetite, vomiting, constipation, diarrhea, duodenal ulcers and other intestinal distress, depression, muscle spasms, arm and leg pain, neuromuscular degeneration, skin problems, cardiovascular disorders, restlessness, respiratory infections, premature aging, kidney problems, loss of hair, weakened adrenal glands, and muscle cramps.

♠ Food sources include meats, organ meats (such as liver), fish, poultry, eggs, milk, cereal, whole grains, legumes, and brewer's yeast.

Vitamin B$_6$ (pyridoxine)

♠ Vitamin B$_6$ is a water-soluble vitamin.

♠ Vitamin B$_6$ is necessary for proper immune function. It is involved in the synthesis of several neurotransmitters and neurohormones (including epinephrine, serotonin, dopamine, and melatonin) and assists in the transport of potassium into the cells. Vitamin B$_6$ is needed for healthy nerves, muscles, blood, and skin.

♠ Signs of a deficiency include insomnia, weakness, fatigue, depression, glucose intolerance, anemia, arthritis, irritability, intestinal distress, skin problems (such as seborrhea, acne, and eczema), hair loss, vomiting, and carpal tunnel syndrome. Prolonged deficiency can result in growth failure, learning disabilities, dizziness, problems in urinating, muscle spasms, impairment of motor function, and, eventually, convulsions.

♠ Food sources include meat, organ meats (such as liver), poultry, fish, fruits (especially bananas), whole grains (including whole wheat and wheat germ), legumes, nuts, seeds, and brewer's yeast.

Vitamin B$_{12}$ (cyanocobalamin)

♠ Vitamin B$_{12}$ is a water-soluble vitamin.

♠ Vitamin B$_{12}$ is needed for activation of folic acid (and vice versa). It is essential for the synthesis of choline, methionine, and nucleic acids, as well as for proper brain, nerve, and red blood cell function.

♠ Deficiency signs include chronic fatigue, skin hypersensitivity, smooth tongue, folic acid anemia, pernicious anemia (characterized by neurological disturbances, muscle weakness, deficit of red blood cells), general weakness, nervousness, problems speaking and walking, and poor appetite.

♠ Food sources include meats, organ meats (such as liver and kidney), poultry, fish, milk, eggs, shellfish, comfrey leaves, bananas, brewer's yeast, kelp, concord grapes, and bee pollen.

Folic acid

♠ Folic acid is a water-soluble vitamin.

♠ Folic acid is involved in the formation of new red blood cells and the synthesis of DNA, methionine (and other amino acids), and choline. It is required for proper cell division, normal neural tube development in the fetus, and synthesis of nucleotides. Folic acid helps maintain a good appetite, improves lactation, and is important for red blood cell formation, body growth, protein metabolism, reproduction, cell division, and hydrochloric acid production.

♠ Signs of a deficiency include digestive problems (such as diarrhea, constipation, and heartburn), loss of appetite, mental depression or confusion,

SECRETS
OF NATIVE
AMERICAN
HERBAL
REMEDIES

214

irritability, insomnia, fatigue, frequent infections, a depressed immune system, anemia (large-cell type), a smooth, red tongue, canker sores, impaired circulation, and growth problems.

♠ Food sources include meat, liver (and other organ meats), eggs, legumes, seeds, whole grains, wheat germ, brewer's yeast, mushrooms, nuts, asparagus, broccoli, lettuce, deep green leafy vegetables, and lima beans.

Biotin

♠ Biotin is a water-soluble vitamin.

♠ Biotin plays an important role in metabolism, glycogen and fatty acid synthesis, and amino acid breakdown. It is essential for the Krebs cycle and energy production, and it fights baldness, arteriosclerosis, alcoholism, high cholesterol, ringing in the ears, constipation, eczema, dizziness, headaches, insomnia, hypoglycemia, and high blood pressure.

♠ Signs of a deficiency include nausea, appetite loss, depression, fatigue, dry skin, hair loss, dandruff, weakness, muscle pain, elevated blood cholesterol, abnormal heart action, and insomnia.

♠ Food sources include egg yolk, milk, organ meats (such as kidney and liver), beef, some vegetables (including cauliflower and mushrooms), nuts, legumes, whole wheat, brewer's yeast, fruit, unpolished rice, and soybeans.

Para-amino benzoic acid (PABA)

♠ PABA is a water-soluble vitamin.

♠ PABA plays an important role in protein breakdown and utilization. It functions in blood cell formation, intestinal health, and skin health. PABA can be manufactured by intestinal bacteria and can stimulate the bacteria to produce folic acid (so it often occurs in combination with folic acid).

♠ Signs of deficiency include digestive distress (such as constipation), fatigue, depression, anemia, loss of libido, headaches, gray hair, and irritability.

♠ Food sources include brewer's yeast, liver, wheat germ, molasses, kidney, whole grains, rice bran, peas and other green vegetables, egg yolk, peanuts, and beans.

Inositol

♠ Inositol is a water-soluble vitamin.

♠ Inositol works closely with pantothenic acid, PABA, folic acid, and B_6. It plays a role in cell membrane integrity and is involved in nervous system function. Inositol occurs in animal tissues as a component of phospholipids and in plant cells as phytic acid.

♠ Signs of a deficiency include constipation, hair loss, eczema, high blood cholesterol, and eye problems.

♠ Food sources include animal foods (as myoinositol), liver, beef brains and heart, whole grains, brewer's yeast, molasses, seeds, nuts, legumes, citrus fruits, raisins, cantaloupe, peanuts, wheat germ, milk, and lecithin.

Choline

♠ Choline is a water-soluble vitamin.

♠ Choline is associated with cholesterol and fat utilization. It acts as a basic component of lecithin (an emulsifying agent) and is essential for the health of the kidneys, liver, and nerve fibers' myelin sheath (the principal covering of the nerve fibers). Choline plays an important part in nerve impulse transmission and is essential for synthesis of the neurotransmitter acetylcholine.

♠ Signs of a deficiency include fatty deposits in the liver, high blood pressure, impaired kidney and liver function, bleeding stomach ulcers, cirrhosis of the liver, fat intolerance, atherosclerosis, and heart trouble.

SECRETS
OF NATIVE
AMERICAN
HERBAL
REMEDIES

216

♠ Food sources include lecithin, grains, egg yolk, liver, legumes, wheat germ, brewer's yeast, and green leafy vegetables.

Vitamin C

♠ Vitamin C is a water-soluble vitamin.

♠ Vitamin C fight infections, diseases, allergies, the common cold, and cancer; it is essential to vascular function, wound healing, bone and joint formation, and red blood cell formation. Vitamin C stimulates the adrenal glands to produce hormones, aids in detoxification, is a potent antioxidant, improves the function of many enzymes, enhances the absorption of iron, assists in converting cholesterol to bile salts, and is required for converting folic acid to its active form and for collagen production.

♠ Signs of a deficiency include anemia, depression, frequent infections, bleeding gums, loosened teeth, muscle degeneration and pain, hysteria, bone fragility, joint pain, rough skin, blotchy bruises, and poor wound healing. Extreme deficiency causes scurvy (marked by bleeding gums, weight loss, anemia, hemorrhages, and muscle and cartilage degeneration).

♠ Food sources include citrus fruits (such as oranges, tangerines, grapefruits, lemons, and limes), rose hips, apples, cantaloupe, strawberries, papayas, guavas, mangoes, black currants, persimmons, dark green vegetables (such as broccoli and turnip greens), red and green peppers, lettuce, tomatoes, potatoes, and cauliflower.

Vitamin D

♠ Vitamin D is a fat-soluble vitamin.

♠ Vitamin D is involved in regulating the transport and absorption of calcium and phosphorus. It play a part in bone formation and resorption, is involved in the process of insulin secretion and the hematopoietic system, and is produced in the skin after exposure to sunlight.

HEALING
MEDICINE
AND THE
POWER OF THE
GREAT SPIRIT

217

♠ Signs of a deficiency include poor muscle tone, restlessness, impaired bone growth, rickets, and osteomalacia in adults.

♠ Food sources include fish oils (including cod liver oil) and oily fish (such as sardines, herring, and salmon); also liver, butter, vegetable oils, egg yolks, and vitamin-D fortified milk.

Vitamin E

♠ Vitamin E is a fat-soluble vitamin.

♠ The vitamin E group includes the tocopherols (alpha, beta, gamma, and delta). Of these, alpha tocopherol is the most active. Vitamin E acts as an intercellular antioxidant, improves circulation, helps resist diseases at the cellular level, and aids in stimulating heart function.

♠ Signs of a deficiency include muscle weakness and wasting, neurologic symptoms (such as poor coordination, cerebellar ataxia, and peripheral neuropathy), anemia, breaking of red blood cells and fragile capillaries, heart disease, involuntary eye movement, sterility, impotence, miscarriages, dull, dry, or falling hair, enlarged prostate gland, tooth decay, gastrointestinal disease, and premature aging. Deficiency is common in those suffering from malabsorption syndromes.

♠ Food sources include vegetable oils, margarine, wheat germ, nuts, seeds, legumes, whole grains, green leafy vegetables (such as spinach), brewer's yeast, Brussels sprouts, soybeans, and eggs.

Vitamin K

♠ Vitamin K is a fat-soluble vitamin.

♠ Vitamin K is important for normal blood clotting. It functions in the formation of proteins containing gamma carboxyglutamic acid (GLA) and activates proteins in the bone and the kidneys.

♠ Signs of a deficiency include ruptured capillaries, easy bruising, impaired bone mineralization, osteoporosis, bleeding ulcers, diarrhea, nosebleeds, miscarriage, increased tendency to hemorrhage, diarrhea, and lowered vitality.

♠ Food sources include green leafy vegetables (such as broccoli, Brussels sprouts, spinach, turnip greens, and kale), kelp, cauliflower, tomatoes, egg yolk, liver, soybean, safflower, vegetable and fish liver oils, and pork.

Vitamin P Complex (flavonoids)

♠ Flavonoids are water-soluble.

♠ Flavonoids are probably best known for their ability to improve capillary strength. Capillaries are tiny vessels that fan out throughout our bodies, supplying nutrients and removing wastes from every cell. When they weaken (a condition known as capillary permeability), nutrients can't get in and waste products can't get out—a traffic jam occurs. Disease and other disasters are just around the corner. Flavonoids are also effective antioxidants and help vitamin C by preserving its action and increasing vitamin C's absorption.

♠ Signs of a deficiency include capillary fragility, bruising, and bleeding gums.

♠ There are more than 2,000 individual members of the flavonoid group, widely distributed in the plant kingdom (especially in vegetables and fruits). They are found in the rind (white pulp) of citrus fruits including oranges, grapefruit, and lemons; in cherries, prunes, apricots, berries (including blackberries and blueberries), in the seeds and skins of red grapes, red wine, and green tea. They are usually found in flowering plants, clover blossoms, buckwheat, soybeans, rose hips, hawthorn berries, black currants, elderberries, peppers, shepherd's purse, horsetail, seeds of milk thistle, plus leaves of the eucalyptus and pagoda tree.

HEALING
MEDICINE
AND THE
POWER OF THE
GREAT SPIRIT

219

MINERALS

Minerals perform a number of roles in the body. Some function as cofactors to our body's enzymes; others regulate fluid and electrolyte balance or provide rigidity to the skeleton. Still others regulate the function of muscles and nerves. Minerals also work together with vitamins, hormones, peptides, and other substances to regulate the body's metabolism.

As with vitamins, we must get our minerals from outside sources (through food or supplements) because our bodies cannot manufacture them. Minerals are found in a variety of foods, but only in limited amounts. In addition, oxalates (found in many fruits and vegetables) and phytates (from grains) may interfere with the absorption of many minerals.

Calcium

♠ Calcium helps build strong bones and teeth and helps us to maintain bone mass as we age. It also plays important roles in muscle and nerve cell function.

♠ Signs of a deficiency include rickets, retarded growth (in children), muscle tetany, neuromuscular overexcitement, osteomalacia, and osteoporosis.

♠ Food sources include milk and other dairy products (such as yogurt, cheese, and cottage cheese), meat, fish, eggs, beans, fruits, and vegetables (especially green, leafy vegetables).

Chromium

♠ Chromium is essential to human nutrition and health and is required for normal carbohydrate, protein, and fat metabolism. We need chromium for proper muscle development, energy production, and blood sugar regulation. A cofactor for insulin, chromium plays a vital role as a glucose tolerance factor.

SECRETS
OF NATIVE
AMERICAN
HERBAL
REMEDIES

220

♠ Signs of a deficiency include impaired glucose tolerance (high sugar diets can increase chromium losses in the urine, as can trauma, stress, pregnancy, infection, and exercise).

♠ Food sources include liver, oysters and other seafood, red meats, chicken, black pepper, cheeses, nuts, whole grains, and brewer's yeast.

Cobalt

♠ Cobalt is a component of vitamin B_{12}.

♠ Because cobalt is part of vitamin B_{12}, a deficiency of this mineral will create a B_{12} deficiency, marked by fatigue, skin hypersensitivity, a smooth tongue, anemia, general weakness, nervousness, problems speaking and walking, and poor appetite.

♠ Food sources include vegetables (including green leafy vegetables), fruits (such as figs), and buckwheat.

Copper

♠ Copper is important in protein metabolism, phospholipid synthesis, and wound healing. It assists in converting iron into hemoglobin and works with manganese in immune response and with zinc to keep the arteries flexible.

♠ Signs of a deficiency include impaired respiration, general weakness, anemia, bone and skin disorders (relating to connective tissue problems), bleeding tendencies, heart disease, an impaired immune system, pancreatic atrophy, and free radical toxicity causing cellular damage.

♠ Food sources include meats, organ meats (such as liver), shellfish (including oysters), nuts, legumes, and whole grains.

HEALING
MEDICINE
AND THE
POWER OF THE
GREAT SPIRIT

221

Iodine

♠ Iodine helps the body to form the thyroid hormones triiiodothyronine (T_3) and thyroxine (T_4), important in regulating energy control mechanisms and cellular metabolic rate.

♠ Signs of a deficiency include goiter (the most obvious sign), cretinism, deaf mutism, and myxedema (a type of swelling often associated with hypothyroidism in adults).

♠ Food sources include iodized salt, seafood, shellfish, cod liver oil, dairy products, and vegetables grown in iodine-rich soil.

Iron

♠ Iron is required for hemoglobin biosynthesis; it is an essential component of many enzymes required for the production of energy in cells throughout the body.

♠ Signs of a deficiency include anemia, lethargy, flatulence, loss of appetite, pallor, and increased incidence of infection.

♠ Food sources include meat, organ meats (such as liver and kidney), shellfish (such as clams), dried fruit, nuts, egg yolk, blackstrap molasses, and legumes.

Magnesium

♠ Magnesium plays important roles in building protein, muscle contraction, nerve function, energy production, calcium assimilation, and bone and tooth formation. It is necessary for glucose metabolism, blood clotting, and synthesis of fats, proteins, and nucleic acid.

♠ Signs of a deficiency include neuromuscular problems (muscle weakness and tremors) and cardiovascular system disorders (irregular heartbeat).

SECRETS
OF NATIVE
AMERICAN
HERBAL
REMEDIES

222

♠ Food sources include milk and other dairy products, nuts, legumes, leafy green vegetables, whole grain cereals, and seafood.

Manganese

♠ Manganese is necessary for normal neural function; protein and carbohydrate breakdown; and fatty acid, cholesterol, and hemoglobin synthesis. It assists in urea synthesis, prevents lipid peroxidation, and activates enzymes needed for vitamin C, biotin, thiamin, and choline use.

♠ Signs of a deficiency include bone abnormalities, carbohydrate and lipid disturbances, growth defects, central nervous system manifestations, reproductive dysfunction, abnormal glucose tolerance, and insulin metabolism.

♠ Food sources include whole grains, nuts, dried fruits, green leafy vegetables, and tea.

Molybdenum

♠ Molybdenum has a role in several metalloenzymes and also in iron metabolism.

♠ Deficiencies in humans are unknown (because necessary amounts are so minute). An excess can cause enzyme inhibition.

♠ Food sources include milk and other dairy products, dried legumes (such as beans and peas), organ meats (such as liver and kidney), and whole grains.

Phosphorus

♠ Phosphorus is necessary for bone and tooth formation, maintenance of acid-base balance, energy production, cell permeability, and nerve and muscle activity. It is a component of proteins, phospho-lipids, nucleic acids, phosphates (buffers) of body fluids, and ATP.

HEALING
MEDICINE
AND THE
POWER OF THE
GREAT SPIRIT

223

♠ Signs of deficiency include poor muscle coordination, fatigue, weight loss, irritability, poor growth, rickets (in children), and gastrointestinal tract dysfunction.

♠ Food sources include meat, fish, poultry, dairy products (such as milk and cheese), eggs, legumes, and whole grains.

Potassium

♠ Potassium is essential for normal growth and maintains proper water balance between body fluids and cells. It is important in nerve transmission, muscle activity, and protein synthesis and works together with sodium to normalize the heartbeat.

♠ Signs of a deficiency include cardiac disturbances and paralysis. Diuretics can increase urinary losses of potassium, leading to a deficiency.

♠ Food sources include whole and skim milk, meat, poultry, fish, whole grains, fruits (including oranges, grapefruit, bananas, prunes, cantaloupe, and raisins) and vegetables (such as asparagus, potatoes, watercress, and peppers).

Selenium

♠ Selenium is essential for some metabolic processes, sometimes acting as an enzyme activator, sometimes as an enzyme inhibitor. It works with vitamin E in its role as an antioxidant.

♠ Signs of deficiency include an increased risk for asthma and chronic conditions (such as cancer and cardiovascular diseases). A deficiency can decrease the activity of glutathione peroxidase in red blood cells; selenium supplementation can increase platelet glutathione peroxidase activity.

♠ Food sources such as organ meats (liver and kidney) and seafood are the richest sources of selenium, followed by cereal and grains, dairy products, and fruits and vegetables.

SECRETS
OF NATIVE
AMERICAN
HERBAL
REMEDIES

224

Silica

♠ Silica is essential for proper growth and development. It plays a vital role in cartilage, collagen, and bone biosynthesis and fights osteoporosis and atherosclerosis. It occurs in nature as silica (silicon dioxide).

♠ Deficiencies have not been produced in man, but with advanced age comes a decreased silicon content in the skin, thymus, and aorta. The level of silicon in the arterial wall decreases with the development of atherosclerosis.

♠ Food sources include whole grain and cereal products, unrefined high fiber, root vegetables, alfalfa, brown rice, beets, horsetail grass, soybeans, leafy green vegetables, parsley, buchu, uva ursi, chaste berry, ginger root, and bell pepper.

Sodium

♠ Sodium works with potassium to normalize heartbeat and helps maintain cellular fluid balance. It aids in maintaining proper blood pH and is involved in muscle contraction and nerve transmission.

♠ Sodium deficiencies are rare (since our diets are usually so high in sodium), but a deficiency can occur because of vomiting, diarrhea, or excessive sweating. A deficiency could cause nausea, muscle cramping, abdominal cramps, confusion, convulsions, and coma.

♠ Food sources include cured meats (such as ham), pork, sardines, cheese, sauerkraut, green olives, and snack foods.

Zinc

♠ Zinc is needed by more than 300 of the body's enzymes. Zinc is needed for white blood cell immune function, wound healing, growth, development, and thyroid hormone function. Zinc works with insulin, interacts with platelets in blood clotting, affects behavior and learning, and is needed to produce retinal (the active form of vitamin A) in visual pigments. Zinc is essential to normal taste, sperm production, and fetal development, and helps protect the body from heavy metal poisoning.

♠ Signs of a deficiency include disturbances in taste and smell, growth retardation, depressed immunity, learning impairment, low sperm count, faulty pancreatic function, insulin reduction, reduced blood-clotting ability, reduced thyroid hormone function, and delayed wound healing.

♠ Food sources include red meats, seafood, wheat germ, legumes, and nuts. Plant sources are less bioavailable than animal sources because of the presence of phytic acid.

ENZYMES

Nothing can exist without enzymes. No plant, animal, or human could survive without these catalysts. During every moment of our lives, enzymes keep us going. At this very instant, millions of tiny enzymes are working throughout your body causing reactions to take place. You couldn't breathe, hold, or turn the pages of this book, read its words, eat a meal, taste the food, or hear a telephone ring without enzymes. Historically, the existence of American Indians was centered around the "magic force of life." We now know that force is enzymes, put here by the Creator.

So far, researchers have identified more than 3,000 different kinds of enzymes in the human body. There are millions of these energizers that renew, maintain, and protect us. Every second of our lives these enzymes are constantly changing and renewing, sometimes at an unbelievable rate.

Fresh, raw fruits and vegetables (and their juices) are rich in enzymes, as are fresh, fermented foods (such as sauerkraut and yogurt) and enzyme "enhancers"—foods usually eaten in small quantities but that pack a big enzyme punch (such as sprouts, raw honey, and wheat germ). Enzymes are also available in supplement form.

SECRETS
OF NATIVE
AMERICAN
HERBAL
REMEDIES

226

See my *Complete Book of Enzyme Therapy* for more information on beneficial enzymes, minerals, phytochemicals, and vitamins.

Exercise

Exercise is the fourth part of the plan. Unlike modern Americans, historically, Native Americans were not sedentary; they used their bodies daily in physical activities such as growing crops, harvesting herbs and other wild plants, tracking, hunting, making their clothing, building their homes, and participating in ritual dances. Physical exercise increases circulation and enzyme activity and helps cleanse the body. American Indian ritual dances are not only good exercise but also are spiritual in nature and heal and cleanse the body. Native Americans believe there is rhythm in nature and that participating in ritual dances can help us get in tune with this rhythm. In this way, one's body will be healthier and have less physical, mental, and emotional stress, and more energy. Native American stomp dances incorporate these rhythms in their sounds, movements, and spirit. These rhythms put one in tune with nature, allowing for a healthier body.

To maintain your health, try exercising six to seven days a week. Walk, bicycle, or swim thirty to sixty minutes a day. If you miss a day or so, exercise the following day, but don't give up. You can do it!

Positive Mental Attitude

The fifth and final part of the plan is a positive mental attitude through meditation, prayer, relaxation, and spirituality. Native Americans, of course, strive to remain balanced. One method is to achieve peace through the ritualistic use of herbs. Herbs and other plants have a soul and a spirit and are used to bless their fellow beings, the humans. The traditional Native American handles plants with great care, always aware of the plant's emotions and feelings, which could be helpful in healing.

HEALING
MEDICINE
AND THE
POWER OF THE
GREAT SPIRIT

227

Herbs are helpful in dream and vision quests and in searching for the balance in life. Knowing and accepting that there is a loving Creator who has given us nature's bounty and who will cure us of our ills can help give us all a positive mental attitude.

As plants unselfishly give of their energies, so must we do the same. We must have total forgiveness for those who may cause us pain and suffering. With this will come a release of guilt, which is blocking a return to health, an inner peace, and the powerful well-spring of energy will be set free from within us.

Consistent self-reinforcement is a good way to improve your mental attitude. Look in the mirror in the morning upon rising, and say at least five times: "I am somebody, God is with me always." For if God, our Creator, is with us, who can be against us?

Nobody!

Take five minutes, twice a day, for quiet time. Find a room where you can be alone. Lie on the floor or sit relaxed in a chair. Rest your hands (palms up) on your lap or at your sides (if lying on your back). Visualize that all the stress is passing from within your body, then feel the stress passing down your arms and feet and out your fingertips and toes. Breathe easily and slowly in through your nose and out through your mouth. Your lips and teeth are parted slightly, and your jaw rests easily. As the air passes out of your mouth, slowly but steadily, utter the word, "p-e-a-a-c-e." Repeat this process as many times as you wish, just visualize (feel) all the stress and pressure leaving your body and allow the inner peace to assert itself.

It is through meditation, prayer, relaxation, and spirituality that we attain a positive mental attitude and total health. See my *Complete Book of Enzyme Therapy* and *Back Pain Bible* for further information on this topic.

Quick Chapter Review

♠ The Creator has placed you on this earth for a purpose and given you all the benefits of nature to heal, clothe, feed, and shelter you.

♠ You can best fulfill that purpose by acquiring and maintaining spiritual, mental, and physical health and harmony.

♠ Illness and injury result from an imbalance and disharmony of the spirit, mind, and body.

♠ The spirit must first be healed before balance can be restored and the mind and body can recover.

♠ For complete healing to occur, forgiveness is essential. Ask the Creator for forgiveness for any past aggressions done to others and forgive those who have offended you.

♠ Only the Creator can heal, but herbs can help maintain balance, harmony, and health. Herbal doctors and medicine men are only channels or tubes of the Creator's healing powers.

♠ Use my Five-Step Jump-Start Program to maintain health and to fight illness or injuries.

♠ When you fall off the path, climb right back on again and continue down the road chosen for you by your Creator. You can do it!

♠ Peace will be with you.

HEALING
MEDICINE
AND THE
POWER OF THE
GREAT SPIRIT

229

APPENDIX A.

Alternative Holistic Health-Care Practitioners

Your general medical practitioner is probably well trained in traditional medicine and quite competent; however, chances are that he or
she has had little training in the use of herbs or in conservative, holistic health care.

If you'd like to incorporate the use of the Native American herbs discussed
in this book into your health-care regimen, you must seek the services of a
well-trained holistic health-care practitioner. Unfortunately, finding one near
you is not always easy. The following organizations should be able to help you
find a qualified holistic health-care provider, including chiropractors, naturopaths, acupuncturists, homeopaths, osteopaths, and others.

The American Association of Naturopathic Physicians
8201 Greensboro Drive #300
McLean, VA 22102
Telephone: (703) 610-9037
Fax: (703) 610-9005
Internet: http://www.naturopathic.org

The American Chiropractic Association
1701 Clarendon Boulevard
Arlington, VA 22209
Telephone: (800) 986-4636
Fax: (703) 243-2593
Internet: http://www.acatoday.com

American Holistic Medical Association
6728 Old McLean Village Drive
McLean, VA 22101
Telephone: (703) 556-9245
Fax: (703) 556-8729
Internet: http://www.holisticmedicine.org

American Osteopathic Association
142 East Ontario Street
Chicago, IL 60611
Telephone: (800) 621-1773
Fax: (312) 202-8200
Internet: http://www.aoa-net.org

American Preventive Medical Association (APMA)
P.O. Box 458
Great Falls, VA 22066
Telephone: (703) 759-0662 or (800) 230-APMA
Fax: (703) 759-6711
Internet: http://www.APMA.net

International Chiropractors Association
1110 N. Glebe Road, Suite 1000
Arlington, VA 22201
Telephone: (800) 423-4690 or (703) 528-5000
Fax: (703) 528-5023
Internet: www.chiropractic.org

International College of Applied Kinesiology
Internet: http://www.icak.com

National Center for Complementary and Alternative Medicine
   Clearinghouse
NCCAM Clearinghouse
P.O. Box 8218
Silver Spring, MD 20907-8218
Telephone: (301) 589-5367 or (888) 644-6226
TTY/TDY: (888) 644-6226
Fax: (301) 495-4957
Internet: http://www.NCCAM.gov

Society of Certified Nutritionists
2111 Bridgeport Way, W, #2
University Place, WA 98466
Telephone: (800) 342-8037
Fax: (253) 566-1851
Internet: www.certifiednutritionist.com

The following resources may be consulted for information on Native American healing:

Association of American Indian Physicians
1225 Sovereign Row, Suite 103
Oklahoma City, OK 73108
Telephone: (405) 946-7072
Fax: (405) 946-7651
Internet: http://www.aaip.com
E-mail: aaip@ionet.net

Freita Kelliche
Ancient Ways of Knowing Foundation
4620 Bradford Heights
Colorado Springs, CO 80906

Telephone: (719) 527-4238
Fax: (719) 527-1649
E-mail: ancientwok@aol.com

Society of American Indian Dentists
P.O. Box 15107
Phoenix, AZ 85060
Telephone: (602) 954-5160

APPENDIX B.

Herbal Suppliers

You can buy American Indian herbal formulas at your local health-food store and many herbal shops. In fast, many larger cities have shops that specialize in American Indian herbal formulas. You can also obtain herbs from the following companies:

Acta Health Products
1131 N. Fair Oaks Avenue
Sunnyvale, CA 94089
Telephone: (415) 459-4393
Fax: (415) 459-4391
Internet: http://www.actapharmacal.com

Aphrodisia Herbs
264 Bleecker Street
New York, NY 10014
Telephone: (212) 989-6440

Bio-Botanica, Inc.
75 Commerce Drive
Hauppauge, NY 11788
Telephone: (631) 231-5522

Bio-Force
4001 Cote Verth
Montreal, PQ H4R 1R5, Canada
Telephone: (514) 335-9393

Brion Herbs Corporation
9250 Jeronimo Road
Irvine, CA 92718
Telephone: (949) 587-1214

Dragon River Herbal
P.O. Box 74
Ojo Calienta, NM 87549
Telephone: (505) 583-2348

Earthrise Company
424 Payran Street
Petaluma, CA 94952
Telephone: (707) 778-9078

Eclectic Institute
36350 Industrial Way
Sandy, OR 97055
Telephone: (800) 332-HERB;

(503) 668-4120

Four Seasons Herb Company
17 Buccaneer Street
Marina Del Rey, CA 90292

Golden State Herbs, Inc.
P.O. Box 810
Occidental, CA 95465

Haussmann's Pharmacy
534–536 West Girard Avenue
Philadelphia, PA 19123-1444

Health Concerns
2415 Mariner Square Drive, #3
Alameda, CA 94501
Telephone: (800) 233-9355

The Herb and Spice Collection
P.O. Box 299
Norway, IA 52318
Telephone: (800) 365-4372

Herb-Pharm
P.O. Box 116
William, OR 97544
Telephone: (541) 846-6262

Herb Products Company
11012 Magnolia Boulevard
P.O. Box 898
North Hollywood, CA 91603-0808
Telephone: (800) 877-3104

The Herb Works
Unit 5, 1007 York Road
Guelph, ON N1E 6Y9
Telephone: (519) 824-4280

Herbs, Etc.
1340 Rufina Circle
Santa Fe, NM 87501
Telephone: (800) 634-3727

Indiana Botanical Gardens, Inc.
P.O. Box 5
Hammond, IN 46325

K'an Herb Company
2425 Porter Street
Soquel, CA 95073
Fax: (408) 479-9118

Kanpo Formulas
P.O. Box 60279
Sacramento, CA 95860
Telephone: (916) 487-9044

Kwan Yin Chinese Herb Co., Inc.
P.O. Box 18617
Spokane, WA 99208

Lorann Oils, Inc.
P.O. Box 22009
Lansing, MI 48909
Telephone: (800) 248-1302

Lotus Light Enterprises
P.O. Box 1008-NW
Silver Lake, WI 53170
Telephone: (800) 548-3824

Mayway Corporation
1338 Mandela Parkway
Oakland, CA 94607
Telephone: (800) 262-9929
www.mayway.com

Nature's Herb Company
1010 46th Street
Emeryville, CA 94608
Telephone: (510) 601-0700

Nature's Herbs
600 E. Quality Drive
American Fork, UT 84003
Telephone: (801) 763-0700

Nature's Way
P.O. Box 4000
Springville, UT 84883
Telephone: (800) 9-NATURE

Nu-Life Nutrition
871 Beatty Street
Vancouver, BC V6P6P2, Canada

Old Amish Herbal Remedies
4121 16th Street N.
St. Petersburg, FL 33703
Telephone: (800) 323-4372

Solaray
1104 Country Hill Drive, Suite 300
Ogden, UT 84403
Telephone: (801) 626-4956

Swiss Herbal Remedies
181 Don Park Road
Markham, ON L3R 1C2, Canada
Telephone: (416) 475-6345

Threshold Enterprises
23 Janesway
Scotts Valley, CA 95066
Telephone: (831) 438-6851

Vita Health
150 Beghin Avenue
Winnipeg, MB R2J 3W2, Canada
Telephone: (204) 661-8386

Wakunaga
23501 Madero
Mission Viejo, CA 92691
Telephone: (800) 421-2998

Winter Sun Trading Company
107 North San Francisco Street, Suite #1

Flagstaff, AZ 86001
Telephone: (520) 774-1501
Fax: (520) 774-0754
Internet: http://www.wintersun.com
E-mail: wintersn@primenet.com

Wyoming Wildcrafters
Wilson, WY 80304
Telephone: (304) 733-6731

Yerba Prima
740 Jefferson Avenue
Ashland, OR 97520
Telephone: (800) 488-4339; (541) 488-2228

Zand Herbal Formulas
P.O. Box 2039
Boulder, CO 80306
Telephone: (800) 800-0405

APPENDIX C.

Sources of Further Information

INTERNET

 The following are some Internet links that may provide more information about Native American healing, herbs, and natural healing, in general.

A Guide to Alternative Medicine Websites
http://www.gemstate.net/susan/linksAmed.htm

Algy's Herb Page
http://www.algy.com/herb/index.html

Association of American Indian Physicians
http://www.aaip.com

Rich-Heape Films, Inc.
http://www.richheape.com

Ayurveda Holistic Center
http://www.ayurvedahc.com

A home page of *A Modern Herbal*
by Mrs. M. Grieve (originally published 1931)
http://www.botanical.com

GardenGuides:Herb Guide
http://www.gardenguides.com

The Healing Pages
http://www.casema.net/~heal/

Healthlinks Healthcare Directory
http://www.healthlinks.net

Homeopathy: How does it work?
Http://ozemail.com.au/~daood/paulc.htm

Nurse Healer
http://www.nursehealer.com

Shirley's Wellness Cafe
http://www.geocities.com/HotSprings/1158

Wellness Web
http://www.wellweb.com

FOR MORE INFORMATION ON HERBAL MEDICINE

American Botanical Council
P.O. Box 201660

Austin, TX 78720

The Herb Research Foundation
1007 Pearl Street, Suite 200
Boulder, CO 80302

HERBAL COLLEGES

American School of Herbalism
1821 17th Avenue
Santa Cruz, CA 95060
Telephone: (831) 476-6377

Blazing Star Herbal School
P.O. Box 6
Shelburne Falls, MA 01370
Telephone: (413) 625-6875
Fax: (413) 625-6972
Internet: http://www.blazingstarherbs.com

California School of Herbal Studies
P.O. Box 39
Forestville, CA 95436
Telephone: (707) 887-7457
Internet: www.CSHS.com

Dominion Herbal College
7527 Kingsway
Burnaby, BC V3N 3C1, Canada
Telephone: (604) 521-5822
Fax: (604) 526-1561
Internet: http://www.dominionherbal.com
E-mail: herbal@uniseve.com

National College of Phytotherapy
3030 Isleta Boulevard, SW
Albuquerque, NM 87105
Telephone: (505) 255-4241

Northeast School of Botanical Medicine
7 Song
P.O. Box 6626
Itachi, NY 14851-6626
Telephone: (607) 564-1023

Southwest School of Botanical Medicine
Michael Moore
P.O. Box 4565
Bisbee, AZ 85603

Sweetgrass School of Herbalism
6101 Shadow Circle Drive
Bozeman, MT 59715-8384
Telephone: (406) 585-8006
Fax: (406) 585-8006
E-mail: robyn@rrreading.com

HERBAL MAGAZINES, JOURNALS, AND NEWSLETTERS

Herbalgram
6200 Manor Road
Austin, TX 78723
Telephone: (800) 748-2617

Herb Companion Press
243 4th Street

Loveland, CO 80537
Telephone: (866) 624-9388

Herb Quarterly
P.O. Box 2626
San Anselmo, CA 94979
Telephone: (415) 455-9540
Fax: (415) 455-9541
Internet: www.herbquarterly.com

Herbs for Health
243 Fourth Street
Loveland, CO 80537
Telephone: (866) 624-9388

InnerSelf
P.O. Box 591
Gulf Breeze, FL 32562
Telephone: (904) 932-7763

Natural Health
70 Lincoln Street, 5th Floor
Boston, MA 02111
Telephone: (617) 753-8900

Organic Gardening
Rodale Press
33 East Minor Street
Emmaus, PA 18098
Telephone: (510) 540-6278

NATIVE AMERICAN MAGAZINES AND JOURNALS

Akwesasne Notes
Kahniakehaka Nation
Akwesasne Mohawk Territory
P.O. Box 366
Rooseveltown, NY 13683-2052
Telephone: (518) 358-3326
Fax: (518) 358-3488
Internet: http://www.ratical.org/akwesasneNs.html
www.slic.com/mohawkna/home.html

The American Indian Review
3 The Homesteads
Hunsdon, Ware
Herfordshire, SG12 8QJ, England
United Kingdom
Internet: http://www.users.globalnet.co.uk

News from Indian Country
7831 North Grandstone Avenue
Hayward, WI 54843-2052
Internet: http://www.indiancountrynews.com

NATIVE AMERICAN VIDEOTAPES

Rich-Heape Films, Inc.
5952 Royal Lane, Suite 254-4
Dallas, TX 75230
Telephone: (214) 696-6916
Fax: (214) 696-6306
Internet: http://www.richheape.com

VIDEOS

Black Indians: An American Story
How to Trace Your Native American Heritage
Native American Healing in the 21st Century
Tales of Wonder—Native American Stories for Children

GLOSSARY

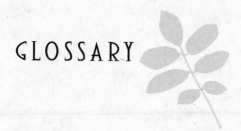

ALTERNATIVE MEDICINE—A broad range of healing philosophies, approaches, and therapies. It is usually not taught in medical schools or used in hospitals. It is also called complementary medicine.

DISEASE—A pathological condition of the body that presents a group of symptoms peculiar to it and that sets the condition apart as an abnormal entity differing from other normal or pathological body states. A medical condition.

DIS-EASE—Literally, dis-ease means a lack of ease, a lack of proper function. A state within a body that exhibits a lack of ease or improper function. A lack of tone within a tissue cell. Also defined as dis-order or dis-function. Dis-ease should not be confused with the medical concept of a disease entity.

EAR CONING—A centuries-old way to relieve earache, to fight infection, and to remove toxins and wax from inside the ear.

GREAT SPIRIT—The Creator who is responsible for the creation of the world. The Great Spirit is recognized in American Indian religious ritual and prayers.

HEALTH—A state of optimal physical, mental, and spiritual well-being and not merely the absence of disease and infirmity.

HERBAL MEDICINE—The use of plant and plant products for pharmacological use. Many drugs commonly used today are of herbal medicine origin.

HOLISTIC HEALING OR HOLISTIC MEDICINE—Therapies in which the health-care practitioner considers the whole person, including physical, mental, and spiritual aspects.

MEDICINE MAN—Native American healers whose knowledge and rituals have been handed down through the centuries. Some medicine people are also shamans, in which case they are often distinguished as holy men and women. The medicine bag, in which they carry their healing secrets, is the symbol of their status and authority.

SWEAT LODGE—A Native American healing and religious ritual, used for purification, spiritual renewal, healing, and education.

TRADITIONAL MEDICINE—Refers to ways of protecting and restoring health that existed before the arrival of modern medicine. These approaches to health belong to the traditions of each country and have been handed down from generation to generation. Traditional systems in general have had to meet the needs of the local communities for many centuries. China and India, for example, have developed very sophisticated systems such as acupuncture and ayurvedic medicine. In practice, the term *traditional medicine* refers to the following components: acupuncture, traditional birth attendants, mental healers, and herbal medicine.

BIBLIOGRAPHY

Mary Dean Atwood, *Spirit Healing: Native American Magic & Medicine* (New York: Sterling, 1991).

——, *Spirit Herbs* (New York: Sterling, 1998).

S. A. Barrett, "Material aspects of Pomo culture," *Bulletin of the Public Museum of the City of Milwaukee* 20, 1952 (92), reprinted as: *Material Aspects of Pomo Culture* (New York: AMS Press, 1980).

Lowell John Bean and Katherine Siva Saubel, *Temalpakh (From the Earth): Cahuilla Indiana Knowledge and Usage of Plants* (Banning, CA: Malki Museum Press, 1972).

Meredith Jean Black, *Algonquin Ethnobotany: An Interpretation of Aboriginal Adaptation in South Western Quebec*, Mercury Series Number 65 (Ottawa: National Museums of Canada, 1980).

Barbara R. Bocek, "Ethnobotany of Costanoan Indians, California, based on collections by John P. Harrington," *Economic Botany* 38(2) (1984): 240-255.

John G. Bourke, *Apache Medicine-Men* (New York: Dover, 1993).

Francis J. Brinker, *The Toxicology of Botanical Medicines*, 2d ed. (Portland, OR: Eclectic Medical Publications, 1996).

Donald J. Brown, *Herbal Prescriptions for Better Health* (Rocklin, CA: Prima, 1996).

Sarah Bunney, ed., *The Illustrated Encyclopedia of Herbs* (New York: Dorset Press, 1984).

C. L. Cantrell, L. Abate, F. R. Fronczek, S. G. Franzblau, L. Quijano, and N. H. Fisher, "Antimycobacterial eudesmanolides from Inula helenium and Rudbeckia subtomentosa," *Planta Med* 65(4) (May 1999): 351-355.

Michael Castleman, *The Healing Herbs* (Emmaus, PA: Rodale Press, 1991).

Ceres, *Herbal Teas for Health and Healing* (Rochester, VT: Healing Arts Press, 1988).

R. Frank Chandler, Lois Freeman, and Shirley N. Hooper, "Herbal remedies of the maritime Indians," *Journal of Ethnopharmacology* 1 (1979): 49-68.

Ranjit Roy Chaudhury, *Herbal Medicine for Human Health*, Regional Publication, SEARO, No. 20 (New Delhi: World Health Organization, 1991).

Barbara A. Chernow and George A. Vallasi, eds., *The Concise Columbia Encyclopedia*, 2d ed. (New York: Columbia University Press, 1989).

Richard Collins, ed., Colin F. Taylor, editorial consultant, and William C. Sturtevant, technical consultant, *The Native Americans* (New York: Smithmark, 1991).

Nelson Coon, *Using Plants for Healing* (Emmaus, PA: Rodale Press, 1979).

Lyle E. Craker and James E. Simon, eds., *Herbs, Spices and Medicinal Plants*, vol. 1 (New York: Food Products Press/Haworth Press, 1986).

——, eds. *Herbs, Spices and Medicinal Plants*, vol. 2 (New York: Food Products Press/Haworth Press, 1987).

——, eds. *Herbs, Spices and Medicinal Plants*, vol. 3 (Phoenix, AZ: Oryx Press, 1988).

——, eds. *Herbs, Spices and Medicinal Plants*, vol. 4 (New York: Food Products Press/Haworth Press, 1989).

John K. Crellin and Jane Philpott, *Herbal Medicine Past and Present*, vol. 2 (Durham, NC: Duke University Press, 1990).

Edward M. Croom, Jr., "Herbal medicine among the Lumbee Indians," in James Kirkland, Holly F. Mathews, C. W. Sullivan III, and Karen Baldwin, eds., *Herbal and Magical Medicine* (Durham, NC, and London: Duke University Press, 1992).

Frances Densmore, *How Indians Use Wild Plants for Food, Medicine & Crafts* (New York: Dover, 1974).

——, *Menominee Music*, SI-BAE Bulletin #102, 1932.

——, *Uses of Plants by the Chippewa Indians,* (1928): 273-379 SI-BAE Annual Report #44 (1928): 273-379.

Nancy Locke Doane, *Indian Doctor Book* (Charlotte, NC: Aerial Photography Services, n.d.).

Dorland's Illustrated Medical Dictionary, 27th ed. (Philadelphia: W. B. Saunders, 1988).

James A. Duke, *Handbook of Medicinal Herbs* (Boca Raton, FL: CRC Press, 1985).

——, *Handbook of Edible Weeds* (Boca Raton, FL: CRC Press, 1992).

David M. Eisenberg, Roger B. Davis, Susan L. Ettner, Scott Appel, Sonja Wilkey, Maria Van Rompay, and Ronald C. Kessler, "Trends in alternative medicine use in the United States, 1990-1997," *Journal of the American Medical Association* 280 (18) (November 18, 1998): 1720.

Thomas S. Elias and Peter A. Dykeman, *Edible Wild Plants—A North American Field Guide* (New York: Sterling, 1990).

Francis H. Elmore, *Ethnobotany of the Navajo* (Santa Fe, NM: School of American Research, 1944).

Charlotte Erichsen-Brown, *Medicinal and Other Uses of North American Plants* (New York: Dover, 1979).

Nancy Evelyn, *The Herbal Medicine Chest* (Freedom, CA: The Crossing Press, 1986).

Mark S. Fleisher, "The ethnobotany of the Clallam Indians of Western Washington," *Northwest Anthropological Research Notes* 14(2) (1980): 192-210.

Hans Flück, *Medicinal Plants* (London: W. Foulsham & Co., 1988).

Steven Foster and Yu Chongxi, *Herbal Emissaries* (Rochester, VT: Healing Arts Press, 1992).

Catherine S. Fowler, *Willard Z. Park's Ethnographic Notes on the Northern Paiute of Western Nevada 1933-1940* (Salt Lake City: University of Utah Press, 1989).

——, *In the Shadow of Fox Peak* (Cultural Resource Series, Number 5, U.S. Department of the Interior, Fish & Wildlife Service, Region 1, Stillwater National Wildlife Refuse, 1992).

David H. Frankel, M.D., "Creating health care," *Hemispheres* (October 1999): 40-43.

Fugh-Berman, "Herb-drug interactions," *Lancet* 355 (9198) (January 8, 2000): 134-138.

Melvin R. Gilmore, *Some Chippewa Uses of Plants* (Ann Arbor: University of Michigan Press, 1933).

——, *Uses of Plants by the Indians of the Missouri River Region* (Lincoln: University of Nebraska Press, 1977).

Rosemary Gladstar, *Herbal Healing for Women* (New York: Fireside/Simon & Schuster, 1993).

A. Grandhi, A.-M. Mujumdar, and B. Patwardhan, "A comparative pharmacological investigation of Ashwagandha and Ginseng," *Journal of Ethnopharmacology*, 44(3) (December 1944): 131-135.

A. M. Gray and P. R. Flatt, "Insulin-releasing and insulin-like activity of the traditional anti-diabetic plant Coriandrum sativum (coriander)," *British Journal of Nutrition* 81(3) (March 1999): 203-209.

Erna Gunther, *Ethnobotany of Western Washington* (Seattle: University of Washington Press, 1992).

Michael Hallowell, *Herbal Healing* (Garden City Park, NY: Avery, 1994).

Paul B. Hamel and Mary U. Chiltoskey, *Cherokee Plants and Their Uses: A 400 Year History* (Sylva, NC: Herald, 1975).

Jeff Hart, *Montana Native Plants and Early Peoples* (Helena, MT: Montana Historical Society Press, 1992).

Jeffrey A. Hart, "The ethnobotany of the Northern Cheyenne Indians of Montana," *Journal of Ethnopharmacology* 4 (1981): 1-55.

Ana Nez Heatherley, *Healing Plants* (New York: The Lyons Press, 1998).

Mathias Hermann, *Herbs and Medicinal Flowers* (New York: Galahad Books, 1973).

James W. Herrick, *Iroquois Medical Botany* (Syracuse, NY: Syracuse University Press, 1995).

I. Hirono, H. Mori, and C. C. Culvenor, "Carcinogenic activity of coltsfoot, Tussilago farfara l.," *Gann* 67 (1) (February 1976): 125-129.

Christopher Hobbs, *Foundation of Health: The Liver & Digestive Herbal* (Capitola, CA: Botanica Press, 1992).

Henry Hobhouse, *Seeds of Change* (New York: Harper & Row, 1986).

David Hoffmann, *The New Holistic Herbal* (Shaftesbury, England: Element, 1990).

K. Hostettmann, A. Marston, M. Maillard, and M. Hamburger, eds., *Phytochemistry of Plants in Traditional Medicine* (Oxford, England: Clarendon Press, 1995).

James H. Howard, *Oklahoma Seminoles Medicines, Magic, and Religion* (Norman: University of Oklahoma Press, 1984).

Hong-Yen Hsu, *How to Treat Yourself with Chinese Herbs* (New Canaan, CT: Keats, 1993).

Judith Benn Hurley, *The Good Herbs* (New York: William Morrow & Co., 1995).

Alma R. Hutchens, *Indian Herbalogy of North America* (Boston: Shambhala, 1991).

Bernard Jensen, *Herbs: Wonder Healers* (Escondido, CA: Bernard Jensen, 1992).

Alex Johnston, *Plants and the Blackfoot* (Lethbridge, Alberta: Lethbridge Historical Society, 1987).

T. K. Jones and B. M. Lawson, "Profound neonatal congestive heart failure caused by maternal consumption of blue cohosh herbal medication," *Journal of Pediatries* 132 (3Pt1) (March 1998): 550-552.

Joseph M. Kadans, *Modern Encyclopedia of Herbs* (West Nyack, NY: Parker, 1970).

John D. Keys, *Chinese Herbs* (Rutland, VT: Charles E. Tuttle Co., 1991).

Kelly Kindscher, *Edible Plants of the Prairie* (Lawrence: University Press of Kansas, 1987).

——, *Medicinal Wild Plants of the Prairie* (Lawrence: University Press of Kansas, 1992).

James Kirkland, Holly F. Mathews, C. W. Sullivan III, and Karen Baldwin, eds., *Herbal and Magical Medicine* (Durham, NC, and London: Duke University Press, 1992).

Claire Kowalchik and William H. Hylton, eds., *Rodale's Illustrated Encyclopedia of Herbs* (Emmaus, PA: Rodale Press, 1987).

Vasant Lad and David Frawley, *The Yoga of Herbs* (Santa Fe, NM: Lotus Press, 1986).

Anna L. Leighton, *Wild Plant Use by the Woods Cree (Nihithawak) of East-Central Saskatchewan*, Mercury Series (Ottawa: National Museums of Canada, 1985).

Walter H. Lewis and Memory P. F. Elvin-Lewis, *Medical Botany* (New York: John Wiley & Sons, 1977).

Y. P. Li and Y. M. Wang, "Evaluation of tussilagone: a cardiovascular-respiratory stimulant isolated from Chinese herbal medicine," *Gen. Pharmacology* 19(2) (1998): 261-263.

S. Lieberman, "A review of the effectiveness of *Cimicifuga racemosa* (black cohosh) for the symptoms of menopause," *Journal of Women's Health* 7(5) (June 1998): 525-529.

C. C. Lin, J. M. Lu, J. J. Yang, S. C. Chuang, and T. Ujiie, "Anti-inflammatory and radical scavenge effects of *Arctium lappa*," *Am. J. Chin. Med.* 24(2) (1996): 127-137.

Lloyd Brother Pharmacists, *Dose Book* (Cincinnati: Lloyd Brother Pharmacists, n.d.).

Richard Lucas, *Nature's Medicines* (North Hollywood, CA: Wilshire Book Company, 1977).

——, *Secrets of the Chinese Herbalists* (Paramus, NJ: Prentice Hall, 1987).

John Lust, *The Herb Book* (New York: Bantam, 1974).

T. J. Lyle, *Physio-Medical Therapeutics Materia Medica and Pharmacy* (London: National Association of Medical Herbalists of Great Britain, 1932).

William S. Lyon, *Encyclopedia of Native American Healing* (New York: W. W. Norton, 1996).

A. R. McCutcheon, S. M. Ellis, R. E. Hancock, and G. H. Towers, "Antifungal screening of medicinal plants of British Columbian native peoples," *Journal of Ethnopharmacology* 44(3) (December 1994): 157-169.

Peter McHoy and Pamela Westland, *Herb Bible* (New York: Barnes & Noble, 1994).

Anne McIntyre, *The Herbal for Mother and Child* (Shaftesbury, England: Element, 1992).

——, *Herbal Medicine* (Boston: Charles E. Tuttle, 1993).

——, *Herbs for Common Ailments* (New York: Fireside/Simon & Schuster, 1992).

Clarence Meyer, *American Folk Medicine* (New York: Thomas Y. Crowell, 1973).

Joseph Meyer, *The Herbalist* (Glenwood, IL: Meyerbooks, 1986).

Charles F. Millspaugh, *American Medicinal Plants* (New York: Dover, 1974).

Earl Mindell, *Earl Mindell's Herb Bible* (New York: Fireside/Simon & Schuster, 1992).

Frank Minirth, Paul Meier, and Stephen Arterburn, *Miracle Drugs* (Nashville, TN: Thomas Nelson Publishers, 1995).

Daniel E. Moerman, "The medicinal flora of native North America: An analysis," *Journal of Ethnopharmacology* 31 (1991): 1-42.

——, *Native American Ethnobotany* (Portland, OR: Timber Press, 1998).

James Mooney, *James Mooney's History, Myths, and Sacred Formulas of the Cherokees* (Asheville, NC: Historical Images, 1992).

Michael Moore, *Medicinal Plants of the Desert and Canyon West* (Santa Fe: Museum of New Mexico Press, 1989).

——, *Medicinal Plants of the Mountain West* (Santa Fe: Museum of New Mexico Press, 1979).

——, *Medicinal Plants of the Pacific West* (Santa Fe: Red Crane Books, 1993).

Lewis Henry Morgan, *The Indian Journals 1859-62* (New York: Dover, 1993).

Daniel B. Mowrey, *Next Generation Herbal Medicine* (New Canaan, CT: Keats, 1990).

——, *Proven Herbal Blends* (New Canaan, CT: Keats, 1986).

——, *The Scientific Validation of Herbal Medicine* (New Canaan, CT: Keats, 1986).

Ada Muir, *Healing Herbs* (St. Paul, MN: Llewellyn Publications, 1993).

Edith Van Allen Murphey, *Indian Uses of Native Plants,* 3d ed. (Glenwood, IL: Meyerbooks, 1991).

J. J. Murphy, S. Heptinstall, and J. R. Mitchell, "Randomised double-blind placebo-controlled trial of feverfew in migraine prevention," *Lancet* 2(8604) (July 23, 1988): 189-192.

Michael T. Murray, *The Healing Power of Herbs* (Rocklin, CA: Prima Publishing, 1992).

Penelope Ody, *The Complete Medicinal Herbal* (London: Dorling Kindersley, 1993).

——, *Home Herbal* (London: Dorling Kindersley, 1995).

Mannfried Pahlow, *Healing Plants* (Hauppauge, NY: Barron's Educational Series, 1993).

Lee Allen Peterson, *Edible Wild Plants* (New York: Houghton Mifflin, 1977).

Mary Summer Rain, *Earthway* (New York: Pocket Books, 1990).

Jeanne Rose, *Jeanne Rose's Modern Herbal* (New York: Perigee Books, 1987).

Penny C. Royal, *Herbally Yours* (Hurricane, UT: Sound Nutrition, 1982).

Humbart Santillo, *Natural Healing with Herbs* (Prescott, AZ: Hohm Press, 1993).

Charles Francis Saunders, *Edible and Useful Wild Plants of the United States and Canada* (New York: Dover, 1934).

Douglas Schar, *Thirty Plants That Can Save Your Life!* (Washington, DC: Elliot & Clark Publishing, 1993).

Paul Schauenberg and Ferdinand Paris, *Guide to Medicinal Plants* (New Canaan, CT: Keats, 1990).

W. J. Simmonite and Nicholas Culpeper, *Herbal Remedies* (New York: Award Books, 1957).

Adelma Grenier Simmons, *The Illustrated Herbal Handbook* (New York: Hawthorn Books, 1972).

Huron H. Smith, "Ethnobotany of the Forest Potawatomi Indians," *Bulletin of the Public Museum of the City of Milwaukee* 7 (1933): 1-230.

——, "Ethnobotany of the Menomini Indians," *Bulletin of the Public Museum of the City of Milwaukee* 4 (1923): 1-174.

——, "Ethnobotany of the Ojibwe Indians," *Bulletin of the Public Museum of Milwaukee* 4 (1932): 327-525.

Gene Spiller and Rowena Hubbard, *Nutrition Secrets of the Ancients* (Rocklin, CA: Prima Publishing, 1996).

Raymond Stark, *Guide to Indian Herbs* (Blaine, WA: Hancock House Publishers, 1981).

Matilda Coxe Stevenson, *The Zuñi Indians and Their Uses of Plants* (New York: Dover, 1993).

Malcolm Stuart, ed., *The Encyclopedia of Herbs and Herbalism* (Leicester, England: Black Cat, 1994).

Gladys Tantaquidgeon, *Folk Medicine of the Delaware and Related Algonkian Indians* (Harrisburg: Pennsylvania Historical and Museum Commission, 1972).

——, "Mohegan medicinal practices, weather-lore and superstitions," *SI-BAE Annual Report* #43 (1928): 264-270.

——, *A Study of Delaware Indian Medicine Practice and Folk Beliefs* (Harrisburg: Pennsylvania Historical Commission, 1942).

Linda Averill Taylor, *Plants Used as Curatives by Certain Southeastern Tribes* (Cambridge, MA: Botanical Museum of Harvard University, 1940).

Deanne Tenney, *An Introduction to Natural Health* (Provo, UT: Woodland Books, 1992).

Louise Tenney, *Today's Herbal Health* (Provo, UT: Woodland Books, 1992).

BIBLIOGRAPHY

263

Robert J. Theodoratus, "Loss, transfer, and reintroduction in the use of wild plant foods in the upper Skagit Valley," *Northwest Anthropological Research Notes* 23(10) (1989): 35-52.

Lalitha Thomas, *Ten Essential Herbs* (Prescott, AZ: Hohm Press, 1996).

Lesley Tierra, *The Herbs of Life* (Freedom, CA: The Crossing Press, 1992).

Michael Tierra, *The Way of Herbs* (New York: Pocket Books, 1990).

T. Tode, Y. Kikuchi, T. Kita, J. Hirata, E. Imaizumi, and I. Nagata, "Inhibitory effects by oral administration of ginsenoside Rh2 on the growth of human ovarian cancer cells in nude mice," *Journal of Cancer Research and Clinical Oncology* 120(1-2) (1993): 24-26.

Traditional Native American Tobacco Seed Bank and Education Program (TNAT), information retrieved from web site http://www.tobacco.org/Misc/tnat.html.

Maria Treben, *Health from God's Garden* (Rochester, VT: Healing Arts Press, 1988).

Nancy C. Turner and M. A. M. Bell, "The ethnobotany of the Coast Salish Indians of Vancouver Island, I and II," *Economic Botany* 25(1) (1971): 63-64, 335-339.

Nancy Chapman Turner and Marcus A. M. Bell, "The ethnobotany of the Southern Kawakiutl Indians of British Columbia," *Economic Botany* 27 (1973): 257-310.

Nancy J. Turner, Randy Bouchard, and Dorothy I. D. Kennedy, *Ethnobotany of the Okanagan-Colville Indians of British Columbia and Washington* (Victoria, BC: British Columbia Provincial Museum, 1980).

Nancy J. Turner and Barbara S. Efrat, *Ethnobotany of the Hesquiat Indians of Vancouver Island* (Victoria, BC: British Columbia Provincial Museum, 1982).

Nancy J. Turner, John Thomas, and Barry F. Carlson et al., *Ethnobotany of the Nitinaht Indians of Vancouver Island* (Victoria, BC: British Columbia Provincial Museum, 1983).

Nancy J. Turner, Laurence C. Thompson, and M. Terry Thompson et al., *Thompson Ethnobotany: Knowledge and Usage of Plants by the Thompson Indians of British Columbia* (Victoria, BC: Royal British Columbia Museum, 1990).

Paul Twitchell, *Herbs the Magic Healers* (Crystal, MN: Illuminated Way, 1986).

Varro E. Tyler, *The Honest Herbal* (New York: Pharmaceutical Products Press, 1993).

H. C. A. Vogel, *The Nature Doctor* (New Canaan, CT: Keats, 1991).

Virgil J. Vogel, *American Indian Medicine* (Norman: University of Oklahoma Press, 1970).

Peter M. B. Walker, ed., *Larousse Dictionary of Science and Technology* (New York: Larousse, 1995).

Carly Wall, *Naturally Healing Herbs* (New York: Sterling, 1996).

J. E. Weaver, *Prairie Plants and Their Environment* (Lincoln: University of Nebraska Press, 1968).

Steven A. Weber and P. David Seaman, *Hevasupai Habitat: A. F. Whiting's Ethnography of a Traditional Indian Culture* (Tucson: University of Arizona Press, 1985).

Michael A. Weiner, *Earth Medicine Earth Food* (New York: Fawcett Columbine, 1991).

Michael Weiner, *Weiner's Herbal* (Mill Valley, CA: Quantum Books, 1990).

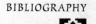

Gaea and Shandor Weiss, *Growing and Using the Healing Herbs* (New York: Wings Books, 1985).

Rudolf Fritz Weiss, *Herbal Medicine* (Gothenburg, Sweden: Ab Arcanum, 1988).

Melvyn R. Werbach and Michael T. Murray, *Botanical Influences on Illness* (Tarzana, CA: Third Line Press, 1994).

Edith Grey Wheelwright, *Medicinal Plants and Their History* (New York: Dover, 1974).

Martha White, ed., *Traditional Home Remedies* (Yankee Publishing, 1997).

Michael R. Wilson, "Notes on ethnobotany in Inuktitut," *The Western Canadian Journal of Anthropology* 8 (1978): 180-196.

John Witthoft, "Cherokee Indian use of potherbs," *Journal of Cherokee Studies* 2(2) (1977): 250-255.

Matthew Wood, *Seven Herbs: Plants as Teachers* (Berkeley, CA: North Atlantic Books, 1987).

H. H. Wustenberg, Henneicke-von Zepelin, G. Kohler, and U. Stammwitz, "Efficacy and mode of action of an immunomodulator herbal preparation containing echinacea, wild indigo, and white cedar," *Adv. Ther.* 16(1) (January/February 1999): 51-70.

Maurice L. Zigmond, *Kawaiisu Ethnobotany* (Salt Lake City: University of Utah Press, 1981).

Index